Reiki

A Key to Your Personal Healing Power

Lena Johansson

LOTUS
PRESS

This book is not intended to treat, diagnose or prescribe. The information contained herein is in no way to be considered as a substitute for a consultation with a duly licensed health care professional.

Library of Congress Cataloging-in-Publication Data
Johansson, Lena
Reiki, A Key to Your Personal Healing Power
ISBN: 0-910261-34-2
I. Subject   I. Title
Library of Congress Control Number: 2001-131265

First U. S. Edition, 2001

Cover, page design and layout: Kerry Jobusch, KPComm

Published by:
Lotus Press
P.O. Box 325
Twin Lakes, Wisconsin 53181
Web: www.lotuspress.com
E-mail: lotuspress@lotuspress.com
(800) 824-6396

ACKNOWLEDGMENTS

*F*irst of all I want to thank my Reiki Master Teachers, John and Esther Veltheim, co-founders of the Reiki Network, for all the knowledge they have so generously shared with me and all their students. A big thanks to Staffan Fritzsche who has spent endless hours helping to translate this book. A special thanks to Brian Olden who proof-read the book and made it grammatically correct. I thank Peter Forster for all his support, joy and love. A humble thank you to all my Reiki students who have shared their lives and their beautiful, unique Reiki stories with me. Thanks to all of you who believed in me and my writing, especially Johnn Donaldson for all the valuable comments. A very special thanks to my father Gœsta Johansson, who kept the fax-communication open and managed to keep all the balls in the air. Each one of you has brightened my life and given me more than I can ever make up for. May joy and happiness accompany you on your journey through life.

TABLE OF CONTENTS

Acknowledgments iii
Introduction vi
1. Background 1
2. What is Reiki? 7
3. The Subtle Anatomy 15
    The Aura 15
    The Subtle Anatomy 16
    The Chakras 21
    Yin and Yang 25
4. Symptoms and Disease 29
5. Beyond the Physical 49
    Opening the Communication with
    the Higher Self 51
    Responsibility 53
    Negative Influence 54
    Masks, Armor and Roles 56
    Manipulation 58
    Change 58
    Freedom of Choice 60
    The Tide of Life 63
    The Observer Within 65
    Detachment 65
    Relationships 67
    Love 68
    Surrender 70
    Living Spiritually 72
    Reiki and Your Power Within 73
6. Reiki Treatments 77
    Treatment of Yourself 77
    Treatment of Others 92
    Children and Reiki 104
    Group Reiki 106

Marathon Reiki 108
When Reiki Appears not to Work 108
7. Other Treatments 113
Treating Animals 113
Treating Plants 114
Food, Drink and Cigarettes 116
Inanimate Objects 118
8. Associations and Training 119
Associations 119
Training 123
Personal Refelections 133
9. People's Encounters with Reiki and Their Own Stories . . . 137
Seminar Information and Orders 153

INTRODUCTION

*R*eiki is a simple, natural, hands-on healing technique that helps in relaxing, releasing stress and maximizing the body's health-potential. Through simple hand-positions the practitioner can treat both himself and others, thereby accelerating the natural healing process of the body. By activating the potential life force in our bodies, we are given access to a harmonious energy that promotes health on all levels: physical, emotional, mental and spiritual. Reiki can be learned during a two-day seminar where the energy is activated to radiate from the hands of the participants at the slightest touch of all living beings.

No previous knowledge is required to learn Reiki. Anyone can use the technique irrespective of age, social standing, religion, etc. When placing the hands on the body the energy is automatically drawn to any imbalances, assisting in the healing process of these areas. The user needs no knowledge of anatomy or physiology since the energy is drawn to the problem without our personal involvement. We are simply radiating the energy once it has been activated in our hands. No extensive training, education or special intellectual capability is required in order to work with Reiki. The attunement process is immediate, and at the end of the seminar the energy flows with full power, equally strong from all participants.

Reiki strengthens the body both physically and psychologically. The consciousness is expanded, the inner awareness is deepened, and creativity, intuition and intellect are stimulated. That is why Reiki is such an effective tool for personal growth and unfoldment. Regular use of Reiki contributes to a sound attitude to life, higher stress tolerance, healthier body and mind, more energy and a decreased need for sleep.

Reiki gives us strength to deal with problems we had previously regarded as insurmountable. It thereby helps us to get on with life. We find it becomes easier to re-assume responsibility for our own life, and actively take charge of our situation. Reiki is an excellent complement to other treatments and techniques, promoting optimal health, development and inner harmony.

This book is for those who are looking for something new and special. That "something" you have known for a long time must exist, but have not yet found. This book is also for those who have already been attuned to the Reiki energy and are using the technique, as well as for those who started but gave up somewhere along the way. It is my hope that you who read this book, whether you are a beginner, a Master or somewhere in between, will be more inspired and reach a deeper understanding of the Universal Life Energy that belongs to us all. The energy which, when attuned according to the Mikao Usui System, is called Reiki.

ONE

BACKGROUND

*T*he word Reiki comes from Japan and is often translated into Universal Life Energy. The Reiki technique does not stem from Japan but from one of our earliest cultures.

According to the Reiki Masters who introduced Reiki to the western culture, Reiki has its roots in Tibet. However, the art of Reiki is probably more than ten thousand years old, whereas the Tibetan culture is only a couple of thousand years old at the most. Therefore, it is not entirely true that Reiki is from Tibetan roots. It is more probable that Reiki has its origins in more ancient cultures, such as the Indian or maybe the Egyptian. It is even theoretically possible that Reiki was used in the most ancient of all known cultures, the Sumerians.

The Sumerians lived on the fertile plains between the rivers of Eufrat and Tigris in what previously was Mesopotamia, and where Iran, Iraq and Syria are situated today. The Sumerians had their era of greatness more than six thousand years ago. Their culture was very advanced and they stood out as very skillful astrologers, amongst other things. They mapped out the entire solar system without the help of telescopes or other technical equipment. Even their trade was well developed and it is believed that it was the Sumerians that invented the sailing boat and the plough. Perhaps the origin, understanding and development of the Reiki technique also stems from the long since extinct culture of the Sumerians. Today we can only speculate about where and how Reiki once began.

Reiki probably spread to Egypt and further north through India, to eventually reach the highlands of Tibet. The knowledge of Reiki was then a well kept secret and well hidden from the lower ranks and classes of society. To receive Reiki was probably very difficult and required many years of preparation and hard discipline. Only certain monks and hierarchy knew about Reiki. Despite the isolation of Reiki the knowledge was spread to China, Japan and possibly elsewhere, through wars and migration.

The modern story of Reiki has to some extent been twisted, through the attempts of wanting to create a legend around the unique method of healing that today is called Reiki. Most of the story has not been possible to verify. A lot in this tale seem to have been created to reinforce the feeling that the storyteller is rendering something legendary. This is the story of Reiki as it has been told, with some variations, since Reiki came into contact with the western culture. Please remember this is just a saga and a skillfully developed legend:

The story starts in Kyoto, Japan, during the Meiji-Dynasty in the 19th century. At this time a man by the name of Mikao Usui was living in Kyoto. It is said he was the principal and a teacher at a Christian school for boys. (We suspect this was said in order to make the technique of Reiki more acceptable in the Americas.) The story continues to tell that Usui's life one day underwent a dramatic change due to his pupils' persistent questioning. It is said Usui's students questioned the scriptures he was citing. These scriptures painted stories of great healers creating miracles through the simple touch of the hand. As Usui admitted he believed these stories to be true his students demanded a practical demonstration. Usui was unable to meet his students request and his humiliation was a fact. This event caused Usui to give up his position in order to seek the answer to this complicated matter. Usui never doubted. He was convinced that earlier cultures had been able to speed up the natural healing process of the body by the simple laying on of hands. He was also convinced it would be possible for the man of today to do the same if only he knew how.

It is said that Usui started his quest for Reiki in the USA, at the University of Chicago. (This is a later addition to the story, possibly to enhance it further. Today it is indicated that Usui never left his home country.) The legend continues that Usui, after many years of theological studies without achieving results, returned to Japan to pursue further research. Usui continued to study Buddhist scriptures where healing by laying on of hands is often mentioned. Usui traveled through Japan and visited temples and monasteries throughout the country asking for more knowledge. He found no one able to help in his quest.

Usui's search eventually lead him back to Kyoto and a small monastery there, where a Zen abbot offered him accommodation. The abbot encouraged Usui to continue his search in the old Buddhist Sutras (teachings). Usui studied these texts, initially in Japanese, but he soon realized that important parts of the message could have been lost in the translations. Instead he began to read the texts in their original language. Usui therefore first learned Chinese to be able to read and interpret the ancient Chinese Sutras, and later he learned Sanskrit the oldest written language in India.

After many years of traveling and searching, Usui eventually found the answer to his long research. It is said he found a formula of mystical symbols in the Lotus Sutras which he understood to be of great importance. Usui sensed the symbols he had found were powerful structures of energy. He realized that when these symbols, or energy patterns, were activated it would be possible to utilize the energy he had been searching for so long. The energy that Usui called Reiki and that in our language has been translated into Universal Life Energy was rediscovered.

The legend says that to understand the full meaning of the symbols, Usui decided to climb the holy mountain of Kuri Yama not far from Kyoto. There he would go through traditional ceremonies of fasting and meditation to increase his awareness, and thereby reach deeper understanding and insight. The legend gives many descriptions of what happened during the twenty-one days Usui spent on the mountain and how he reached his insights.

It is said Usui achieved a form of heightened awareness where he experienced a deep understanding of the dynamics of Reiki. When Usui regained his wakened state of consciousness he experienced a new, powerful energy in his hands. He knew that he had found the energy that he had been searching during so many years. Usui's walk back to the monastery has been the basis for many more or less credible stories.

When Usui reached the monastery, he and the abbot agreed that Usui would need to test the effects of Reiki. To do so Usui moved to the outskirts of the city where the poor and the sick were living in the so called "Beggar Kingdom". There he tried to gain a deeper understanding of Reiki and its efficiency by helping the sick and disabled.

According to the legend Usui stayed in the "Beggar Kingdom" for seven years. Then he started to travel through the country, this time to spread the knowledge of Reiki, give treatments and attune the energy in others. He continued his travels in Japan for many years.

In 1920 Usui met Chujiro Hayashi, a 47 year old reserve naval officer and doctor. Hayashi would become a dedicated student of Usui. He also became one of the successors of Reiki after Usui's death in 1926. Hayashi opened a clinic in Tokyo where he and many of his Reiki students successfully treated sick people. One of the first Reiki clinics had been founded.

The legend now takes us to the island of Hawaii in approximately 1933. Here lived a young, Japanese woman holding American citizenship. Her name was Hawayo Takata. She was a young widow left with two small daughters. Takata was in very poor health, suffering from colon cancer, gall stones, inflamed appendix and other disorders. During a trip to Japan Takata was told about the Reiki clinic. She was curious and decided to try this unknown form of treatment, instead of going through with previously planned surgery. Within five months of daily Reiki treatments her illnesses and problems were gone. Furthermore, Takata had been convinced that she wanted to dedicate her life to working with Reiki. After three weeks of treatments she was also attuned to Reiki. Later Hayashi trained Takata to the Grand Master level and named her one of his successors. They both agreed that she would take over the Reiki clinic in Tokyo after Hayashi's death.

In 1937 Takata completed her training with Hayashi. Hayashi helped Takata establish Reiki in Hawaii and they also gave some Reiki seminars together.

Hayashi died in 1940 and Takata traveled to Japan to be present at his death. Thereafter she returned to Hawaii to get her belongings. She was now going to settle in Japan to continue Hayashi's work at the clinic in Tokyo. But the Second World War forced Takata to stay in Hawaii. Japanese Americans had a very difficult time during the war and their freedom of movement was drastically limited. She had to wait for the end of the war before she was once again permitted to travel freely and could return to Japan.

Takata went back to Japan to resume Hayashi's work. On her return she found that the entire area had been totally destroyed by bombs. It is said that the only building that had not been destroyed by the war was the Reiki clinic. Hayashi's widow had converted the clinic into a refuge for homeless, young women. The two women decided the widow should continue to run the shelter while Takata returned to Hawaii.

Takata established Reiki in Honolulu where she continued to give Reiki treatments and initiate islanders in Reiki for more than thirty years. Much later she was invited to the mainland to give a First Degree Reiki Seminar. This became something of a turning point both for Takata and for Reiki, since the demand for Reiki turned out to be very great. Many people wanted treatments, and several more wanted to learn how to use Reiki themselves. During the 1970s Takata traveled the United States and Canada giving Reiki seminars and training more Reiki Masters.

Hawayo Takata was a very powerful and charismatic woman. At this time her name started to become widely known outside the borders of North America, even as far away as Australia and Europe. Takata trained twenty-two Masters before her death in 1980. Regardless of the opinions of some of these Masters and others, Takata did not officially name any particular one of them as her immediate successor. Instead she left the responsibility with each individual Reiki Master to go out in the world and spread the knowledge of Reiki. Many new Reiki Masters have been trained since Takata's death and several new Reiki associations have been established in different parts of the world. You will find more information about different associations and the levels of education in chapter 8.

Today there is an ever growing interest in Reiki in the Western culture. Soon this simple, natural method for healing of the body and mind will be as accepted as many of the alternative therapies we are already using today. Known methods such as massage, chiropractic and acupuncture were treated with great skepticism a number of years ago, but are accepted in most areas of society today. The applications for Reiki in the future has a scope far beyond its uses of today, particularly as a complement to conventional medicine.

The simplicity of Reiki is amazing and makes it suitable for everyone. Reiki is an excellent aid, for healing active illnesses as well as for preventive health care. Reiki is an easy method for self-help that will become far better known in the very near future.

TWO

WHAT IS REIKI?

*R*eiki is a simple, natural and harmonious energy with powerful healing abilities. The energy is activated in the body by a very simple attunement technique, during a two-day Reiki seminar. As a result of the attunement, the hands start to radiate harmonious energy whenever touching any living organism. The practitioner simply places his hands on his own or somebody else's body allowing the energy to flow. Reiki balances unhealthy vibrations and imbalances in the energy systems of the body supporting the body's own healing process.

In order to explain what Reiki is and how it works, we first have to find and answer to what energy is. Energy has various meanings to different people. I will try to explain the term energy and how Reiki, as an energy, works.

Energy comes in many forms, for example, as the food we eat to gain strength to get through the day, or as electricity produced from sun, wind, water, oil and nuclear power that we use for lighting and heating. Energy moves in endless cycles. It can never be destroyed, only transformed into other forms of energy. Static (potential) energy can be transformed into kinetic energy that can be transformed further into thermal energy. Picture the water in a dam as potential or static energy which is transformed into kinetic energy when it is let through the dam gates and rushes down wards. The water runs through special turbines where the kinetic energy is transformed into electricity. It is possible to produce electricity from the water since the water contains potential energy.

There are many forms of energy in the universe. If we allow ourselves to study our environment we will soon realize that everything around us consists of pure energy: The chair we sit on, the food we eat, and even our own bodies.

Energy is an expression of frequencies, vibrations or waves at different speeds. Energy moves in waves, i.e., in cycles per second. We use Hertz as a measure of cycles per second. Some energies have very slow movements. If the energy in the atoms have very low kinetic energy they form molecules that are very strongly attached to each other. In that way solid matter is formed. The composition, speed and kinetic energy of atoms and molecules varies and therefore different solid forms, objects and beings are created.

The human body is a creation of pure energy. From the outside we appear to be built-up of muscles, organs, bones, blood, etc. but when looking closer it is possible to see that every part of the body is made up of cells. These cells are built of molecules that in turn consist of atoms. Quantum physics tells us that the particles that make up the atomic structure consist of pure, vibrating energy. The human being is a unique energy system, built-up of the smallest parts of the atoms, the sub-atomic particles.

The body not only consists of the physical parts we can feel and touch. In, and around, the body there is also a more subtle anatomy made up of thoughts, feelings, previous conditioning and experiences. These energies create different frequency fields that form distinct "layers" around the physical body. These energy layers are sometimes called the etheric body or Aura. Scientists call these fine energy layers bioplasm. We cannot see or touch the Aura, but most individuals are sensitive enough to feel these energy vibrations in other people. We often "know" how somebody feels before they tell us. If we enter a room full of people, we know if the group has just laughed at a good joke or just ended a stormy argument, without talking to anybody. The emotional energy still lingers in the room and around each individual. Furthermore, our language is full of expressions reflecting this phenomenon. For example: "I could feel it...", "I sensed that..." and "It is in the air...". You can read more about the subtle anatomy and the Aura in chapter three.

Every cell in the body emits a frequency, a small micro vibration, that is reflected in the energies around the physical body. These different frequencies build a tightly knit web of energies, each pulsating in its own speed but in total harmony with the others. In a completely healthy human being the energy systems work without disturbances or imbalances, but that is quite unusual! It is much more common that the individual has disturbances in his subtle energies. This is mainly due to each individual's inability to listen to the body's needs. Man often seems to push himself far beyond his body's physical and mental abilities creating disharmony along the way.

The universe with all its galaxies and solar systems consists of an infinite number of frequencies, all vibrating at different speeds. The wave motions produced are polarized, i.e., the cycles of the wavelengths move between plus and minus, up and down, in oscillating waves. The slower vibrations form solid matter, for example rocks, cliffs, wood, colors and living organisms of different kinds, whereas more subtle frequencies move faster than the eye can perceive. Thoughts and feelings within the body are examples of these rapid vibrations, and so are microwaves, gamma rays and X-rays. Some frequencies move faster than the speed of the light, at what is called supra luminal speed. These frequencies move so fast their polarity seem to disappear. The vibrations are so high that it is impossible to measure any plus and minus charges. These frequencies can only exist in very subtle energy dimensions and they are said to be "unpolarized". In the universe there is no stagnation and even the so called unpolarized energies vibrate, but so fast it can be considered negligible.

Quantum physicists of today are showing considerable interest in the subtle energies creating the subatomic particles. The entire universe is made of atoms, including everything around and inside us. Subatomic particles, that vibrate at an incredible speed, circulate within and around the atoms. Some physicists think that these particles have an intelligence of their own. These particles vibrate at a very high frequency, and some scientists call them "the glue of the universe". Their purpose is to hold our concept of the world together, and they move throughout the universe. They work as a glue that links atoms and molecules together. These miniscule particles are necessary to keep the universal order, and to preserve life in the form we are used to. This particle energy prevents us, and our surroundings, from dissolving. Without this fantastic energy system, the entire universe would collapse and nothing would look like it does today.

The scientists call the phenomenon "The Unified Field Theory". The energy itself is called quanta or Hawkin's energy (after the well-know quantum physician, Stephen Hawkin). Others call the energy cosmic or universal energy. Sometimes it is called Life Force, and it exists within all of us, mainly as a potential energy. Most people have lost the ability to utilize this energy and to use what should be our birth-right: The ability to fully access the ever present Life Force to achieve a stronger body, more energy and increased vitality.

Since Reiki has made its entry into society, there is a possibility for everyone to awaken the subtle Life Force energy within. We can expand and balance our being in harmony with the Life Force energy. The process is called attunement, or initiation, of Reiki. After the attunement process the individual immediately gains increased access to the vibrating Life Force energy. This ability stays for the rest of one's life. The attunement process activates the body to draw from an energy with very strong healing properties. An energy that radiates from the hands when touching living creatures or organic matter. The technique to access this universal life energy is called Reiki.

Reiki has no limitations, and can be used on everything and everybody at any time. The universe consists of Life Force, constantly penetrating and flowing through the body. When the body is attuned to utilize this Life Force we have immediate and infinite access for the rest of our life. Reiki can never be depleted. There is always more, no matter how much we use. In fact, the flow is enhanced the more we use our Reiki.

Reiki is an unpolarized energy that vibrates many times faster than the speed of light. Reiki strengthens the body by recreating balance, and harmonizing distorted energies in the body systems. That way the body's own healing process is enhanced. The body has an extraordinary ability to heal when given the chance. By using Reiki the period of healing can be cut down to half of the normally expected time, and in some cases only a third of the estimated time is necessary in order for the body to get well.

When using Reiki a high vibrational and harmonious energy is transferred to the body from the hands. The energy speeds up the healing at all levels: Physically, emotionally, mentally and spiritually. It is very easy to learn how to use this harmonious form of energy.

However, Reiki cannot be learned from books or tapes, and the ability is not activated by receiving treatments. Reiki is a potential energy that must be activated in the body by a Reiki Master trained in the special technique required. Reiki is not an intellectual knowledge but the result of participating in a two-day First Degree seminar. The attunement process is performed in four steps where the body is gradually accustomed to, and tuned into, the new higher vibrations. By these four different attunements all participants are given the ability to use Reiki for the rest of their lives without limitations.

Reiki is as much a complement to medical care as a method to prevent future health problems. Anybody can learn this technique. No previous knowledge is required. Age and state of mind are of no importance. Small children, very ill individuals and people in comas have all successfully received Reiki.

Every individual body contains a limited amount of life energy which varies with how we feel. The energy level is low when we are tired, worn-out or ill. If we feel well, are healthy, strong and full of life, the energy level is high. Healers in the east have known of the Life Force energy within the body for many thousands of years and they call it Chi or Qi (Ki). Scientists in the west have quite recently "discovered" this subtle, but highly tangible, polarized energy radiating from the physical body, and it can be measured with the help of sensitive electromagnetic instruments.

The human being is very dependent on the level and state of the Chi energy. When we live well and healthy we re-fill our energy storage. Unfortunately we often live our lives in such a way that we deplete our supply of energy faster than we are able to replenish it with nourishing food, exercise, good sleep and enjoyable recreation. Sooner or later this results in fatigue, premature aging and dis-ease. With the help of Reiki we can replenish our energy resources and promote health and vitality on all levels.

Reiki creates harmony in the body's imbalanced energy systems and replenishes the depleted energy resources. We do *not* use our own Chi energy when we give ourselves or somebody else a Reiki treatment. We utilize the vibrating Life Force of the universe, an inexhaustible source of vitality and health beyond the body's own limited energy storage. When giving a treatment to somebody else we also receive Reiki since the energy flows through our own body creating a "spin off" before continuing through the hands into the client. Consequently, we will be more energetic after giving a treatment than before. This is a unique characteristic of Reiki.

Another unique characteristic of Reiki, acquired by the attunement process, is the ability to treat ourselves. We can help heal our own body and prevent future diseases and problems without the risk of depleting our Chi energy.

These characteristics are unique to Reiki! In other forms of healing, that preferably is not to be confused with Reiki, the results can be the opposite. There is a great risk that somebody who does not have Reiki, and who is practicing the laying on of hands, drains the energy from his own body when treating others. Therefore, he is only able to give a limited number of treatments during a set time period. He is not able to treat himself in case he would get sick, and there is a risk that his body will weaken over the years as a result.

Reiki is an energy science. Whether you believe in Reiki or not is irrelevant to its efficiency and results. A Reiki treatment accelerates the body's own healing process by strengthening and balancing disturbances in the body's energy systems. Reiki does not belong to any religion, cult, sect or other faith. Reiki creates optimum healing conditions in the body by restoring harmonious energy. After the attunement process the hands automatically radiate Reiki, irrespective of our own conditionings and belief systems. Furthermore, Reiki is independent of social status, age, frame of mind etc.

The practitioner's own state of health is not important to the strength of the treatment, since an energy beyond the physical body is used. Even seriously ill people radiate energy as strongly as healthy, vital individuals. This has been shown, for example, when cancer patients or people with AIDS or HIV have successfully treated each other with Reiki.

Reiki differs substantially from other forms of healing because it is totally independent of our own health. We can treat ourselves, and receive a spin off of the energy when treating others. All these properties make Reiki a unique form of treatment suitable for everybody.

SUMMARY
- Reiki is a harmonious, balancing energy radiating from the sub atomic particles.
- Reiki accelerates the healing process of the body.
- Reiki replenishes exhausted energy resources of the body.
- Reiki works independently of faith or religion.

- The Reiki energy is inexhaustible.
- Reiki is independent of the practitioner's health.
- You can treat yourself with Reiki.
- No lengthy training or education is necessary in order to use Reiki.
- Once attuned, the ability to use Reiki remains for the rest of your life.
- Reiki expands the awareness and improves intellect, intuition and creativity.
- Reiki is "un-polarized" energy.
- Reiki is preventive health care, as well as a method to help heal the body.
- Reiki maximizes the health potential and increases the quality of life on all levels.

THREE

THE SUBTLE ANATOMY

THE AURA

As well as consisting of physical blood, flesh and bones the body also emits a network of subtle energies invisible to the naked eye. These energies create several high frequency layers around the body. The frequency of these energies increases with every layer. Scientists call this external energy-field, or subtle anatomy, bioplasm. According to old Eastern cultures this energy-field is called the Aura, a name that is also commonly used in the West.

The Aura plays an important role in our health. It reflects who we are, our personality, and how we choose to react or respond to different situations in life. It is in the Aura that previous experiences and conditionings are reflected, expressed as memories and emotions in the physical.

Normally the Aura extends about 10 to 12 inches from the body. It is often contracted, and it can at times be weak and low in energy, depending on the state of the body and how we currently regard ourselves and our situation. During the Reiki attunements the Aura expands dramatically. The four attunements strengthen the Aura and create a permanent expansion of seven to nine feet. The attunements heighten awareness and create an increased sensitivity to the body's demands, and what the human being needs in a larger context. This transformation on a spiritual level is reflected in the expansion of the Aura. We gain clarity in how to treat ourselves and what to do to improve our situation. Stress and exhaustion are thereby lessened.

When the Reiki energy is activated the ability to intuitively understand what could be changed in a situation to achieve a greater well-being is increased. The secret behind this breakthrough is the attunements which expand and strengthen the Aura. By understanding yourself on a deeper level you will find new and unique opportunities and solutions to your problems. You regain strength to take charge of your own life. Further, this will lead to accelerated development. To understand that it is *you* and nobody else that has responsibility for your own situation opens unexpected opportunities, and it is only with this insight and understanding you can start to grow as a human being.

The human being is a complex composition of energies. Around the body there is an invisible field of energy, the Aura. This subtle anatomy strongly affects the body and the general state of health. Usually we believe the body is only what we can see and touch, but in reality there is much more. The ability of the human being stretches far beyond the limited understanding of the mind, just like the universe stretches far beyond what we see when looking up at the sky on a clear and starlit night.

THE SUBTLE ANATOMY

The Aura consists of many different layers or subtle energy bodies. First there is a thin layer of energy that surrounds the physical body just like an invisible body stocking. This layer is approximately one inch thick and it is called the Supra-physical body. The physical energy flowing back and forth through the acupuncture meridians (the energy highways of the body) is reflected in this subtle body. In a healthy body the energies move freely without hindrance from any blockages. Unfortunately it is very common today that people have disturbances and blockages in their energy flow, making them unable to utilize their energy fully. These people constantly feel tired, worn down, stressed and even burned out. This finally manifests in different forms of symptoms and varying degrees of serious diseases, and can eventually lead to the death of the physical body.

The next subtle body is egg-shaped, and surrounds the physical and the supra-physical bodies. This energy-layer is often called the Astral or emotional body. The Astral body reflects all the emotions we hold inside ourselves. Everything from joy, hope and love, to anger, sorrow and hatred, and many, many more. It is extremely important that we learn to recognize and work through the charged emotions experienced during the day, otherwise they will be suppressed and stored in the body. With time this will cause blockages and disturbances, not only in the subtle emotional energy layer but also in the physical body. All of the subtle energy-bodies are closely associated with the physical body, and strongly affect it in positive or negative ways. That is why it is so important that the emotional body is in balance, and that we are in emotional harmony with ourselves and our environment. All the subtle energy bodies are linked through different energy centers called Chakras, and the physical body functions are strongly affected by their existence and degree of harmony.

The next subtle energy-layer is called the Causal body. It too is egg-shaped, and surrounds the Astral body. The Causal body reflects past events, everything we have ever experienced, whether forgotten, suppressed or still in conscious memory. The Causal body also stores the energy of the present, everything occurring in this very moment. It also reflects all the infinite numbers of a person's possible futures.

People do *not* have one fixed destiny ahead of them! Something that inexorably pulls them from one event to another. We are each very unique beings with our own minds and complete free will. The choices we make today will without a doubt create our tomorrow, just like the choices we made yesterday have created the reality we live in today. We cannot blame anybody else for the situation we have put ourselves in, just as we cannot pretend that we have no control over our tomorrow.

You have total responsibility for where, what and who you are, and you can choose to change your situation at *any* time. How you experience life depends entirely on the attitude you have towards the precious and unique experience that is *your* life. So do not give this responsibility away to others. There is no need to see psychics, clairvoyants, mediums or channellers. You have all the knowledge within!

Predictions come true as the medium sees and presents one of the more possible futures of all the infinite numbers of futures you have. Through focusing, more energy is put into that possible future. Afterwards you will continue to put more and more energy into that particular future. Either you add positive energy full of expectations, if you have learned something exciting and fun, or you feed it with negative energy if you have learned something that scares you and that you definitely do not want to experience. In both cases your focus will add more fuel to this particular future. The chance that the prediction will come true becomes many times increased. This pattern is the same as when you work with affirmations to change something in your life or about yourself, by positively focusing on the new "set up" you desire. Using affirmations is a special technique where you influence your subconscious mind towards a positive change, in contradiction to allowing *others* to rule your life. The latter is to give up your free will and the responsibility for your own life. You will soon feel that you have lost control. This will lead to lower self esteem and a feeling of having lost the ability of managing your life. To some people predictions seem to rarely or never come true. These are often powerful people with a high self esteem and a great ability to create their own future. They know what they want and what life to live. They will not let outer circumstances or other people's suggestions interfere with the life-plan they have created.

Everybody can, at any given time, choose to accept a greater responsibility for the life they lead and for the shape it will take. Reiki enhances the ability to listen within to find the answers needed, rather than listening to somebody else.

The egg-shaped energy-layer surrounding the Causal body is called the Mental body. It reflects the conscious mind; all the logic, intellect, reasoning and thinking that constantly goes on in the brain.

The Etheric body is a very thin energy-layer around the Mental body. It reflects the superconscious mind and is represented by parts of the brain that are not consciously used.

The subconscious and superconscious minds are called the unconscious mind, but there is a large difference between the two. The subconscious mind, reflected by the Causal body, stores all previous and future experiences. Ideas, attitudes, beliefs, conditionings and prejudices that we have developed or accepted from those around us at early age are stored here. These belief systems might be totally inappropriate by the time we have grown up. Despite this, as adults, most of us still carry limiting thoughts about ourselves and our world.

The superconscious mind however, plays a totally different role. If you learn how to listen intuitively, this higher aspect of yourself will guide and help you make right decisions on your path through life. The superconscious mind, via its connection to Soul, contains all knowledge and wisdom. It has a total overview of your person and your life-plan. If you learn to listen to your superconscious mind you will be able to walk through life with greater ease and joy.

Reiki strengthens your connection to the superconscious mind and Soul and thereby enhancing your intuitive knowledge. Reiki puts you in contact with the superconscious part of yourself, where all universal wisdom is stored. The superconscious mind is reflected in the Etheric body.

In some literature the term Etheric or ether body is used as a collective name for the energy layers of the Aura. This is in contrast to the Etheric body as the name of one of the outer layers of the Aura. Sometimes the Supra-physical body is called the Etheric body. The reason for the varying names of the energy layers of the

Aura is that they originally stem from different schools of thought or doctrines. The names of these energy layers are not that important. The importance lies in our understanding of the energy bodies' existence, and what they represent in the physical body.

Swirling around the Etheric body are endless numbers of high frequency energy-bodies. These are the Spiritual bodies or Soul bodies. These Spiritual bodies reflect Soul in Its beauty. Soul has all the answers drawing from past experiences for future challenges, and It is constantly communicating with the conscious mind (the ego) via the superconscious. It is therefore important to nurture this connection, and to let the intuition flow, to be aware of the messages coming through. The more blockages, the more difficult it will be to grasp the guidance given, and the harder life will be as the ability to listen within has been lost.

People's Auras are constantly mingled. On a higher level we are all connected and we constantly influence each other's energies. On a subconscious level you are infinitely aware of all the misery, starvation and distress in the world, in the same way as you are affected by the harmony and joy that others experience at this moment, no matter where they dwell. Sometimes it might seem that we have already lost the battle to save the world, but that is but an illusion. At this very moment you have the ability to change the world, by giving of yourself in a positive way. It is high time, but not too late, to regain responsibility for our planet and its development, by starting to change ourselves. Now is the time for as many of us as possible to strive in a positive and harmonious direction. This will be impossible as long as we do not experience balance, strength and harmony within ourselves.

Every time you give yourself a Reiki treatment you will automatically go into a deep, relaxed state where total peace and harmony prevail. The harmony you experience within will spread throughout the world via the fine threads of energy that link all living beings. In other words, you can spread harmony and peace into the world by giving yourself love and nurture. Through the insights you

may receive during or after the Reiki treatment you will gradually
understand the meaning of total harmony, and thereby also the
meaning of peace on earth. You have no right to change somebody
else but through you changing, those around you will gradually
change. Your inner change will slowly spread over the world like
rings on the water. Changing yourself is a genuine way to change
the state of the world from one of hostility, selfishness, war and
misery to one of peace, understanding, harmony and love.

THE CHAKRAS

From deep within the physical body, and through all the subtle layers of the Aura, swirl seven major energy centers. They are
called the Chakras. The word Chakra has its origin in Sanskrit, an
ancient language of India. It means "wheels of spinning energy".
Today the word Chakra is the most commonly used also in the
Western parts of the world.

In the body's fine energy systems there are more than 360
Chakras of different sizes. They are spread throughout the body.
There is for example, one small Chakra in every joint. The body's
seven major Chakras are the most important for now. They strongly affect different bodily functions and interact to a large extent
with the personality.

In each Chakra there is a seat of consciousness represented by
the different emotions held there. The human being expresses the
personality through these emotional energy-centers. Each Chakra
represents different characteristics; the tendency is therefore to under
or over stimulate any of the seven major Chakras, depending on
our personality. Over or under activity of one or more of the
Chakras will eventually lead to imbalances, not only in the subtle energy bodies but also in the physical body.

Each major Chakra influences one each of the seven major
endocrine glands, i.e. hormone producing glands. Each Chakra also
affects one of the seven major nerve complexes in the body. If there
are imbalances in the subtle energy centers, there will eventually

be imbalances in the physical body. Pathological changes in both the glandular system and the nervous system will follow. A well working endocrine system and nervous system are vitally important to the health. It is impossible to stay fully healthy with imbalances in one or the other.

Each major Chakra has its own origins in the body. They affect different organs, endocrine glands and nerve complexes, and each of them portray different characteristic traits. By tradition each Chakra is also represented by one spectral color and by one tone in the harmonic scale.

THE FIRST CHAKRA—THE ROOT CHAKRA

The first major Chakra has its origin in the spinal cord, at the tip of the tailbone. It represents grounding and stability, and the ability to stand with both feet on the ground—to be rooted. The root Chakra deals with how well we adjust to society regarding maintaining ourselves, paying bills, going to work etc. It deals with materialism and how well we manifest the material necessities of life. This Chakra is called the survival Chakra. It is here the control mechanism for "fight or flight" is located. The emotion affecting the first Chakra is fear.

Blockages in the root Chakra can arise if we consider ourselves defenseless victims of circumstances, and thereby have difficulties taking responsibility for ourselves and our situation. You and nobody else has the responsibility for your own maintenance and performing your daily tasks. By daring to live life with all its risks, and by accepting responsibility for each choice and action, you create a better foundation for a well balanced and vital root Chakra.

Physically the root Chakra controls the functioning of the kidneys. The endocrine glands affected are the adrenals. The color for the root Chakra is red, and the tone is C.

THE SECOND CHAKRA—THE SACRAL CHAKRA

The sacral Chakra is located four fingers below the navel, originating from the spinal cord in the lower lumbar area. It influences sexuality and sensuality. Physical love and personal relationships are governed by the second Chakra. How well we develop sensuality and sexuality has nothing to do with the number of partners we go through. A frantic changing of partners shows imbalance in the sacral Chakra. In self-hatred the ability to love and trust in somebody else have been lost, due to belittling and despise of oneself. Acceptance of, and a greater respect for, one's own body strengthens the sacral Chakra.

Physically the sacral Chakra affects the bodily fluids, the urinary tract, the genitals, and the reproductive organs. It is not uncommon that incest or exposure to other sexual violations will create problems with the reproductive system. The active endocrine glands here are the sexual glands (the gonads). The color for the sacral Chakra is orange, and the tone is D.

THE THIRD CHAKRA—THE SOLAR PLEXUS

The solar plexus Chakra is located in the spinal cord, roughly in level with the diaphragm. The third Chakra deals with personal power, independence and vulnerability. The solar plexus Chakra is the prime center for our emotions. It is here the processing and assimilation of all our experiences in life occurs. Anger, hostility, rage, free will and ambition are emotions located in this Chakra. Blockages in the third Chakra are common, since many people have problems claiming their own space and accessing their inner power.

Spleen, stomach, liver and gall-bladder are affected by how we deal with these emotions. The endocrine gland affected by the solar plexus Chakra is the pancreas. The color for this Chakra is yellow, and the tone is E.

THE FOURTH CHAKRA—THE HEART CHAKRA

The fourth major Chakra is located in the middle of the sternum at the level of the nipples, originating from the spinal cord. The heart Chakra holds love, compassion and harmony, and it deals with issues of Soul. It handles unselfish and unconditional love

beyond the little ego's limitations and prejudices, both regarding ourselves and others. Unconditional love is shown when giving of
ourselves without ulterior motives or expectations of receiving in
return. Closing the heart in self hatred, depreciation and disgust, from
fear of being hurt in love, to withdraw into one's own self, stop giving, impatience and stress, all create blockages in the heart Chakra.

Physically the heart Chakra regulates the heart, the blood, the
lungs and the circulatory system. It influences the entire endocrine
gland system, and above all it strongly affects the immune system.
Giving love and compassion to oneself and others strengthens the
immune system and keeps us healthier and more resistant to diseases and infections. Self-hatred and low self-esteem, may eventually
lead to immunological diseases of different kinds. Increased acceptance and compassion of oneself are of vital importance regarding
diseases such as rheumatoid arthritis, HIV and AIDS. The thymus
is the endocrine gland particularly affected by the heart Chakra.
The color for this Chakra is green, and the tone is F.

THE FIFTH CHAKRA—THE THROAT CHAKRA

The throat Chakra originates in the cervical vertebrae at the
level of the vocal cords. It deals with the ability of communication
and expressing oneself. Criticism and judgment are also traits located in the throat Chakra. Blockages arise through self denial and the
inability to communicate ones needs. Many shy and timid people,
who have difficulty speaking up for themselves, have imbalances
in their throat Chakras. As a consequence they may develop problems in the throat and bronchi area. If you have trouble with the
fifth Chakra think of what has not been said. Are you withhold-
ing the truth, or are you assaulting others with the spoken word?
What has been said in a far too angry and harsh way?

The fifth Chakra physically affects the vocal cords, the
bronchial apparatus and the alimentary channel. The metabo-
lism is also regulated here. The endocrine glands affected by the
throat Chakra are the thyroids. The color for this Chakra is blue,
and the tone is G.

THE SIXTH CHAKRA—THE THIRD EYE OR BROW CHAKRA
The sixth Chakra originates in the brain in level with the forehead, in between the eyebrows. It represents intuition, imagination and idealism. The third Chakra is active when manifesting inner dreams into physical reality. Through the third eye you are able to see the more subtle things in your environment. It is possible to train and develop this inner vision to, for example, see Auras around living creatures. Remember though, that such an ability is just a phenomena, a performance act that might keep you stuck in your own ego. Your most important task in life is to learn to see yourself the way you really are! Blockages in the third eye Chakra appear as an unwillingness to see the reality you live in, and can manifest as poor eyesight or in extreme cases even blindness.

The sixth Chakra affects the autonomous nervous system. The endocrine gland affected is the pituitary gland. The color is indigo, and the tone is A.

THE SEVENTH CHAKRA—THE CROWN CHAKRA
The crown Chakra has its origin in the brain, in level with the posterior fontanel. It deals with higher spiritual values, Soul's journey, and the divine quest. The seventh Chakra handles issues beyond our linear space/time understanding and limited minds. Its main purpose is the search and the understanding of our true spiritual purpose on earth.

The crown Chakra affects the central nervous system. The gland affected is the pineal gland. The color is violet, and the tone is B.

YIN AND YANG
Each Chakra contains a positive or negative electromagnetic charge. This has nothing to do with "good" or "bad", but is entirely about electricity. The three lower Chakras; root, sacral and solar-plexus, are positively charged or *Yang* influenced. According to old Eastern wisdom the Yang energy represents masculine, positive, active, extrovert, determined and expansive energy, manifestation and intellect. This positively charged masculine

energy represents the left hemisphere of the brain with its linear and logical thinking. Being grounded, sexuality and personal power are Yang inspired impulses.

The three upper Chakras; throat, third eye and crown, have a negative charge or Yin energy. According to Eastern wisdom, the Yin energy represents feminine, negative, passive, introvert, withdrawn and submissive energy. Characteristics such as sensitivity, spirituality, clairvoyance and intuition are Yin influenced. The Yin energy affects the right hemisphere of the brain with its lateral thinking. The feminine Yin energy has the ability to hold several contradicting concepts simultaneously without conflict. This ability is sometimes condescendingly referred to as female logic, but is indispensable for the social and technological development of mankind. Every successful scientist, man or woman, has a well developed ability to actively use the feminine, intuitive right hemisphere of the brain.

The heart Chakra is neutral and without electrical charge. The task of the loving heart is to unite and balance the negatively charged upper Chakras and the positively charged lower Chakras. It is through unconditional love our masculine and feminine aspects are balanced, both inwardly and outwardly. It is not always easy to create a well functioning and harmonious relationship with a partner as long as there is no balance and love in the inner relationship with oneself. Relationships are however one of the most powerful ways to expand and grow beyond our own limitations, to finally find this inner harmony.

The masculine and feminine energies within have nothing to do with being a man or a woman. For a complete balance both men and women need equal parts of Yin and Yang. Men cannot live in harmony solely by expressing their masculine aspects, such as taking charge and expanding themselves carelessly, using sexuality without integrity, aggressively striving for promotion, etc. They would also need to express respect and consideration, and learn to tap into their Yin inspired intuition, spirituality, creativity and care.

It is not possible for women either to live merely through their Yin energy. They too would need to express masculine characteristics in a harmonious balance with their female energies.

An individual with a Yin/Yang imbalance will attract a partner who physically expresses the lacking or deficient energies. For example, the very masculine macho-man will most possibly attract an extremely feminine woman. In their appearances they both carry what the other one lacks. This kind of relationship is not built on true love and understanding but on a compulsion to fill inner deficiencies and needs through another person. A relationship like this builds on dependency. It creates unrealistic demands and expectations. The chance to achieve a long-lasting, loving and happy relationship under these circumstances is not good. The mutual expectations become insurmountable, and the one is never able to fulfill the other's bottomless needs. To experience a happy relationship we must first create harmony within ourselves. Through understanding of our own needs and functioning, by watching the mirroring in our fellow beings, we will be able to reach a balanced relationship between the male and female aspects within. When this is done, the automatic attraction of a loving partner occurs in perfect harmony. We need that inner realization before we can experience a relationship built on genuine love and trust.

The physical body reflects inner mental and emotional disturbances. Each Chakra is a seat of consciousness. The human being expresses himself through the Chakra system. It is therefore important to understand its existence and characteristics. Be aware of which of the Chakras you use when expressing yourself, and which ones you neglect due to the personality you developed. Unknowingly you have taken part in creating problems with your health and your situation by over or under activating certain of the major Chakras. This will also have affected the endocrine glands and nervous complexes that are connected to these particular Chakras. Your task is to slowly change your personality towards a more balanced existence and subsequently a healthier body, through increased understanding, knowledge and awareness.

The Chakras are constantly exposed to negative influences that create imbalances in the system. In a sick or worn-out body the Chakras most certainly spin at different speeds and in disharmony. It is important for the health to regularly reestablish balance in the Chakra system. Each Reiki attunement realigns the Chakras and reinforces the balance of the system. The four attunements received in the First Degree Seminar cause each Chakra to double in size and spin at the same speed. The entire Chakra system is momentarily in balance. Each time we give ourselves a Reiki treatment we reinforce that balance. The treatments work most effectively if done every day. Reiki is a very efficient technique with which we can influence the body's state of health, simply by creating harmony and balance in the subtle anatomy. Reiki makes us more aware of our constant interactions with our surroundings, and the games we play to fulfill our internal needs. That insight creates strength and contributes to change.

Apart from the seven major Chakras, there are several hundred minor Chakras in the body. Each and everyone of them is linked to one of the major Chakras. The two minor Chakras important when using Reiki are found in the middle of each palm of the hand. The hand Chakras are directly linked to the heart Chakra. It is with the hands we express the love and care flowing from the heart. Furthermore, the hands are our working tools. It is therefore very natural to activate Reiki in the hand Chakras. It is however possible to attune any of the minor Chakras. This might be necessary if somebody lacks one or both hands. In a situation like this it would be most appropriate to attune the minor Chakras in the feet. These individuals will then be able to treat both themselves and others using their feet.

The Chakras play an important role in how we feel, and how we act or react. To experience optimal physical and mental health it is important to understand the role the Chakras play in the body systems, and to actively work for their balance. Reiki is a very special technique developed to create inner and outer harmony. We achieve the best results if we allow ourselves the benefit of Reiki daily.

FOUR

THE BODY'S SYMPTOMS AND DISEASES

*T*he body is made of vibrating energies, i.e., subatomic particles pulsating at different frequencies. The cells forming bones, organs and tissues in the body are made from the elements. These elements spring from an infinite number of minuscule energy particles creating the atoms. The atoms are put together into different molecular structures forming building blocks united into the vast complexity of organs and tissues that create the human body. The infinitesimal particles making the atoms are vortexes of vibrational energy. In reality this means that all matter; solids, liquids and gases, consist of pure vibrating energy. The solid human being is actually made from pure energy.

As man is composed of pulsating energies, each cell emits a measurable micro vibration reflected in the energy field around the body. In composition with the reflections of emotions, memories, experiences, thought patterns, conditionings and belief systems these frequencies form an interconnected web of energies around the body. In a healthy body the energies pulsate at different speeds, but in total harmony with each other. If an imbalance would occur in any of these frequencies the energies closest to the distorted frequency would also be affected and caused to vibrate in disharmony. This means that the distortion will gradually spread through the aura, from frequency to frequency, finally penetrating the body where a physical symptom would occur. This simplified explanation roughly describes the development of various diseases. An illness in the body is merely expressing a *symptom* of an inner imbalance among the subtle energies. Usually this physical

29

symptom is caused by emotional or mental disharmonies of some kind, i.e., thought patterns, feelings and belief systems that negatively affect the bodily functions.

It takes roughly three to four years for the subtle imbalances to reach the physical body and cause a symptom to appear. In some cases the process can be longer. Sometimes it takes half a lifetime or more to develop a particular illness or symptom. In other cases the process can be much quicker, depending on the level of awareness, type of disturbance, and mental state of the individual.

All our previous experiences are stored as conscious or unconscious memories in the brain. These experiences are also locked in the physical body as energy blockages and inflexibilities. Deeply rooted, often suppressed, painful memories and traumas are often stored in the bone structure. Other difficult experiences may be stored in muscle tissues, while more recent experiences of the day are stored in the skin appearing as lines and wrinkles. Suppressing unresolved conflicts and traumas in the body creates inflexibility, bad posture, diffuse pains and premature aging. The chest contracts and the breathing becomes shallow. The more of these unresolved issues that are held within, the more hunched-up and weighed down the body becomes.

Working on earlier conflicts in life can bring about dramatic changes in looks, posture and health. Dissolving and releasing of suppressed and charged memories and emotions stored in the body can create an enormous relief. We feel lighter, regain a straighter posture and a more supple, free and flexible body. Facial lines are smoothed out as the external look becomes more relaxed. The breathing becomes deeper and more released. Pain in joints and muscles decreases or disappears. The body may change by the pure act of remembering, recognizing and facing past traumas. In this process Reiki offers an invaluable tool. Reiki helps the body to let go of its excess luggage by carefully bringing light and understanding to suppressed emotions and experiences involved.

Suppressed memories and emotions are one of the main reasons for the bad health and lack of vitality that many people experience today. If we disregard our problems and refuse to recognize the feelings that are brought about by a certain situation, the charged emotional energies will be stored in different parts of the body. A surplus of suppressed emotions creates very tangible, negative changes in the body. The Chakra system is negatively affected and hence the endocrine system and the larger nervous complexes in the body. In severe cases lumps and tumors may grow, due to excessive amount of accumulated, confined emotional energies. Daily, an enormous amount of energy is used in continuing to suppress these emotions and keeping the internal turmoil under control. If these "forbidden" emotions were released the energy we need to keep them at bay could be used to live our lives with greater strength and vitality.

Each individual has the possibility and capacity to release suppressed energies by recognizing the emotions experienced during the day rather than clenching teeth, pretending the emotion does not exist. It is possible to learn how to work with releasing suppressed emotions by using different methods, where Reiki stands out as a very effective technique. It is important to balance the emotional energies in the body before diseases develop and Reiki works on that level. A combination of Reiki and other body therapies, such as for example Rolfing, Heller Work, Rosen Therapy and Rebirthing, have shown good results in releasing suppressed emotions and physical pain.

In the East, the connection between mind and body has been common knowledge for thousands of years. According to Chinese Medicine, different emotions have special correspondence to different organs and tissues in the body. Therefore, an organ will be affected with greater intensity by the particular emotional energy stored there. This book only deals with this emotion/organ correlation on a superficial basis. If you want a deeper understanding I suggest you look for books specifically written for Acupuncture and Chinese Medicine.

Chinese Medicine is based on the theory that blockages are created in the body when enough of a particular emotional energy has been suppressed and stored in that area. This occurs if we do not have the opportunity, strength, or ability to see, understand and express the emotion at the time it is experienced. If we deny these emotions a natural expression we will in time become walking volcanoes ready to explode at any moment. The "volcanic eruption"can occur in any form, from a sudden inexplicable emotional explosion to a complete nervous break-down. It can also be expressed in different symptoms and various diseases.

Diseases do not fall from the blue. We have often worked quite hard, and for a long period of time, to bring forth the imbalances in the body. Various kinds of accidents are other outlets for suppressed emotional energies to manifest their own release. If there is an imbalance at the subtle energy level, some areas of the physical body will eventually develop blockages and weaknesses. These areas are more apt to injuries than areas of strong healthy and balanced energy. To establish equilibrium, we may attract the accident required to restore balance in the system. This is the body's own security system of indicating the imbalances that later might lead to serious illness if not attended to in time. In very severe cases, if the suppressed emotions are neglected too long, the final expression might be the death of the physical body.

When all else fails, the subconscious mind tries to communicate with the conscious mind by creating diseases and accidents. Via the body it tries to wake us up to the fact that we somehow lead an unhealthy life. The illness or accident shows that we need to re-evaluate our way of living and maybe change some destructive habits. If we were not to develop these diseases we would continue to run the body down to the point where it could no longer keep functioning. There is therefore no reason to hate, deny or despise illnesses. At times they play an important role in the survival of the body. A disease, or the convalescence after an accident, often leaves time to slow down, rest and regain strength. It also offers time for introspection and Soul searching. If we use this time wise-

ly a lot of understanding, change and growth may occur. Seriously
ill people that have regained their health have sometimes changed
their life situation entirely, leading a freer and happier life than before.
This may occur even when the accident or disease caused serious
damage to the body. A new joy and appreciation for life often
replaces the damaged part of the body. This inner joy may in a greater
perspective lead to a longer life filled with deeper meaning and more
satisfaction.

A special medical system based on the connection between the
emotions and the well-being of the body was developed in China
several thousand years ago. The system is called "The Theory of
the Five Elements" and is based on Traditional Chinese Medicine.
This system clearly shows the complexity of the human being.
According to this theory all emotions can be sorted into one of five
basic emotions, each corresponding to one of the five elements: Wood,
fire, earth, metal (air) and water. Each element influences different
organs and tissues in the body, which acts as a storage facility for
suppressed emotions. An excess of suppressed emotional energy will
affect the body pathologically if left without outlet, whereas a
healthy emotional expression will lead to balance and strength. By
working with suppressed emotions their energy is released, and it
is easier to experience the vitality that each organs' psychological
qualities offer. The good psychological characteristics of the organs
play an important role in our daily lives, where they supply common sense, judgment and an enhanced ability to make decisions.
At this level it is most important to be aware of suppressed emotions in excess since they affect the body pathologically. Note that
so called negative emotions act as a positive drive in our daily living as long as they are not in excess, and that the so called positive
emotions may be harmful for the body if expressed excessively.

The Theory of the Five Elements and their Organ Correspondences:

1) ANGER—FURY, RAGE, FRUSTRATION, IRRITATION
     Affects: liver, gallbladder, shoulders, muscles, immune system
     Balancing emotion: kindness

Psychological qualities: control, decisiveness
Element: wood

Every day we experience frustrating and irritating situations. Uncooperative children when late for work, the long line at the bank during lunch-break, red traffic-lights on the way to an important meeting, and all other buttons that are pushed daily. If we are stressed and over-worked, anger and frustration is easily provoked by family members, fellow employees, friends or even total strangers. You may for example observe yourself the next time you are driving in heavy traffic...

Each time we are unable to react constructively to a situation, the subtle energy from the emotions awakened is suppressed and stored, especially in the particular organs and tissues mentioned. After many years of suppressed, denied anger and frustration the stored energies may condense into matter. Gall-stones may be an example of this. There are probably very few people that have never experienced feelings of impotent irritation and anger. Many meet these emotions several times a day. Naturally not everybody will develop problems with gall-stones. We are all individuals with our own experiences, genetic configurations and personalities. This also means that we react with different degrees of resistance to what the body is exposed to. Many people express their inhibited aggressions by developing headaches and migraines for example. The suppressed emotional energies then follow the gall-bladder meridian through the stomach up to the neck and head, where they explode in excruciating pain. In sever migraine attacks with nausea, the body tries to rid itself of the stored "gall"(anger) by throwing up. Other manifestations of these energies are frozen shoulders and painful muscles.

2) FEAR—FRIGHT, TERROR, DREAD, STRESS
Affects: kidneys, bladder, lower back, central nervous system, reproduction, endocrine gland system, knees, ankles
Balancing emotion: gentleness

Psychological qualities: ambition, willpower
Element: water

The evolution of man is very slow. The instinctive reactions of the body are still very similar to those of the cave man. In a threatening situation the body still reacts by producing adrenaline to increase muscular activity and physical strength. This reaction makes it possible to fight in defense in a more effective way, or to quickly run away from a fearful situation. The difference is that today we don't have to fight dinosaurs or saber-toothed tigers. Instead, the threats and aggravations experienced often seem to appear from within, leaving us incapable of dealing with the situation by physical action. The energy produced by the experienced emotion will instead be contained in the body. In the long term this repeated cycle of unexpressed emotional turmoil is very damaging to the body.

A person of today has completely different fears to fight compared to the rough times experienced as a caveman. The fears experienced nowadays mostly deal with how we see ourselves and our situation. The greatest fear most of us hold is the fear of being inadequate. We fear we are not good enough. We fear being a failure unable to live up to expectations and demands put upon us. Often these sometimes impossible expectations are made by ourselves—for ourselves. And woe betides us if we do not live up to the demands we have created. Nobody is as harsh and as judgmental, or criticizes as hard, as oneself when judging one's own appearance and actions. We condemn ourselves to a life in constant fear of not being able to live up to all the demands put upon us by ourselves and society. This fear is very damaging to our health. The more fears we experience and suppress, real or imagined, the more problems we will have with our health. On an energetic level the kidneys, lower back, etc. are affected. The region from the hips downward represents the ability of daring to take the next step forward in life. The pelvic area equates to the support we experience or lack in our present situation. If we are paralyzed with fear it is impossible to make any progress, and we cease to develop in a healthy way in all aspects of our lives.

The knees reflect the ability to muster will-power in different situations. Many times this will-power helps overcome fear in scary situations. We may experience fear but through the power of will we are able to conquer the resistance, move ahead and perform, despite the fear that is trying to hold us back. We need a powerful will to be able to cope in society but sometimes it can be too strong, turning into stubbornness, inflexibility, obstinacy, pig-headedness and refusal to give in. These characteristics in excess interfere with the body's energy balance and can eventually lead to physical symptoms or accidents. If you have problems with your knees, think about what fears you might be dealing with in your life, or if you have developed a too stubborn and unyielding personality.

The ankles express the stability and balance we presently experience. If we find ourselves in a difficult situation that requires a vital decision, it is important not to be paralyzed in agony over this decision. A distortion in the energy around the ankles may develop, and if we are paralyzed for too long, incapable of action, the risk of injuring ourselves in that particular area is increased many times. Sprained or broken ankles are very common, and sometimes the injury is caused in the most surprising way. I have met a number of people who have sprained or broken their ankle during an easy walk on level ground. Often a little pebble or a soft slope is the only visible reason for the accident. The physical conditions of the ground have really nothing to do with the accident. It is the internal hesitation and inability to take a firm stand that creates the increased risk for injuries. It is much more important to our health that we make a decision at all, rather than it having to be the absolute "right"decision. We might not see it at the time of the decision but we are often given the opportunity to correct an earlier choice if we later realize it could have been made differently. During the process of deciding and realizing the outcome of our choice we have probably learned more about ourselves and experienced a period of unfoldment and growth. If we stand still, not daring to choose or go forward in life, we also stop developing and growing as human beings. We freeze in our present life situation, allowing the ever dynamic and perpetual life to run us over.

3) WORRY—ANXIETY, APPREHENSION, NERVOUSNESS
   Affects: stomach, spleen, pancreas, wrists
   Balancing emotions: fairness, openness, honesty
   Psychological qualities: ability to integrate, stabilize, feeling of being centered and balanced
   Element: earth

Too much worry and anxiety often causes a stressed stomach, acidity, gastritis and in more severe cases, ulcers. It was the drive for survival that made apprehension and worry a necessary part of the human race. These feelings call forth a moment of reflection, preventing us from throwing ourselves into dangerous situations without previous consideration. Nowadays though, people worry in excess compromising their health in the process. We worry about practically everything we do. We worry about what might happen "if", "when" or "in case", long before anything at all has happened. We continue to worry while living the situation apprehended, rather than putting our energy into finding a solution to the problem. After the experience we worry about what we might not have done "correctly", or we are concerned about what different outcome we might have caused had we acted in this or that way instead.

Most of what we are worried or anxious about in life will never occur! We waste enormous amounts of energy on all the "ifs" and "maybes" that will actually never take place. The only result from all this worrying is a lower energy potential in the present situation. As a consequence we might experience problems with the stomach or any of the other organs affected by the worry energy. We are simply draining our Life Force energy by all this unnecessary worrying.

Learn to live in the moment! All you have is the infinite now. This present second. And that is all you will ever have. Make this precious moment of your life the best that you possibly can! Nothing will change for the better worrying about a future event that may never occur.

When you find yourself in an anxious event, actively look for solutions rather than getting stuck in numbing trepidation. After the time of distress is over more worries will lead nowhere. What is done is done, and the only thing to do now is to rest assured that you did your very best considering the circumstances. More worry will not change what has been done in the past. In none of these stages will energy put into worry and anxiety give any advantages, whether it is worry before, during or after an incident. On the contrary, worry, anxiety and nervousness will lead to internal imbalances and blockages draining our capacity. From long-term worry the internal energy imbalances created may lead to symptoms and illnesses in the physical body.

4) GRIEF
Affects: lungs, large intestine
Balancing emotions: righteousness, courage
Psychological qualities: strength, substantiality
Element: metal (air)

Grief is a healthy emotional expression that our technological and mechanistic society, to a large extent, forced the modern man to suppress. In many situations we are not permitted to express what and how we feel due to unwritten social "laws". The human being is fundamentally a creature of a rich and active emotional life. Conscious and unconscious attempts to curb and push aside these natural emotional reactions will lead to internal imbalances, blockages and diseases.

As with all emotions, grief must have its outlet. Men and women alike must allow themselves to actively express the grief they experience. The mourning after somebody leaves us through death, divorce or for any other reason must be allowed to take its time. The loss of a loved one may take many years to work through. The more we suppress this process, the longer it will take. Modern society has very little compassion for this. We are allowed to grieve for a certain time but when "the official mourning period" is over we are supposed to have pulled ourselves together, being ready to continue with our lives as if nothing ever happened. But grief goes deeper than this. A person in mourning may feel the need to cry many months or years after the event. The reasons for this can be many or none but a feeling of loss and sadness. A photo, a song on the radio, an idle word, a memory, or simply an urge to cry may get us started. We often cut off this need to express the depth of our being, since it is not so acceptable to cry in public. We restrain the urge, waiting for another occasion to cry, an occasion that may never occur. Instead we bury the tears and grief deep inside the body. Too much pent up grief with no outer expression may manifest as different physical symptoms. If we deny ourselves our tears it is very probable the body will try to express its grief internally. Problems with the lungs, e.g., asthma, pneumonia or edema are not uncommon. Fluid and mucus in the lungs are the body's own way of expressing its internal tears. There are cases in medical history telling of severe lung diseases where the medications and treatments were of no help until the underlying reason, the suppressed grief, was attended to.

It is not only the loss of a loved one that brings about grief and sorrow. Every larger change provides the cause of meeting the end of the old. The known and safe in life are exchanged for new and unexplored territories. We are going through a period of experiencing the death of that which has been, and the feelings of loss must be lived through and expressed. Tears are a healthy outlet for all grief.

5) Joy—sadness, melancholy, depression, impatience
    Affects: heart, circulation, small intestine
    Balancing emotions: love, honor, respect
    Psychological qualities: warmth, vitality, excitement
    Element: fire

Unlike the grief felt when losing someone or something specific the fire element deals with chronic sadness and lack of joy in life. Life is simply not fun any longer. The motivation is lacking and everything seems to move in the same tracks as always. Spontaneous expressions of joy have slowly suffocated in the struggle for survival. There are many occasions through life where we might feel the need to question the purpose of our existence, asking ourselves why we go on at all. Unresolved conflicts in everyday situations and a general dissatisfaction with life can cause sadness, melancholy and depression. Long and drawn out sorrow and depression creates heartache. The heart is bleeding when denied to express joy and laughter and the digestive process of the small intestines deteriorate. People who take life too seriously, the so called A-type personalities or workaholics, run a high risk of developing problems with clogged arteries and heart conditions.

The heart is also harmfully affected by impatience and haste. The human being is not born to rush between different commitments without taking time to fulfill his or her own physical, mental and spiritual needs. Man was not meant to selfishly walk over others on the way to the top of promotion and recognition. People who are grasping without sharing, who selfishly keep others away from what is theirs to avoid someone else getting more than themselves, have closed their hearts and live in disharmony. They have stopped giving of themselves and the warmth they once had. They no longer have patience with those around them. They live in an ego-centered world with no compassion for others. They hurry through life without seeing its beauty. Rushing through life this way diminishes the joy of experiencing togetherness and the feeling of closeness and warmth from others. These individuals no longer support one another; instead they unmercifully sacrifice others in their quest to fulfill their own lives. People leading this kind of life have failed to understand that isolating oneself only leads to emptiness and inner dissatisfaction. The more they strive to become the best, to earn the most money, receive the most fame and recognition, the more hollow they will become in their hearts. They have not yet realized that by giving of themselves to others they will keep their integrity, still attaining everything they have ever strove for and more. The negative influence on the heart leads to all kinds of heart conditions such as cardiac arrest and myocardial infarction, which is so prevalent in today's society.

Even joy in excess may cause too great a strain on the heart. An example could be a person with an already weakened heart who receives some sudden, unexpected but happy information, maybe that he has won five million dollars in a lottery. The joy might be so overwhelming that the heart collapses.

As adults it is important to reclaim the right to our own emotions. Despite the fact that as children we might have learned how to contain anger, fear, grief, sorrow and other emotions, sometimes with cookies and sweets as a bribe. It is possible, however, to learn how to deal with the emotions arising, craving attention, rather than stuffing ourselves with chocolate and cakes. The pattern that has been repeated generation after generation can be broken. We can teach both ourselves and our children to constructively express emotions experienced during the day. It is possible to take an active part in the emotional healing by creating external changes to our situation in life. If we consider ourselves unable to change a particular situation, it is still possible to learn how to search internally for our inherited strength and joy. Simply change the attitude to whatever it is that is causing the sadness or depression. Remember, Soul, your true inner self, is always happy!

The five basic emotions and their correspondence with the organs reflect the problems, symptoms and diseases that may develop if we deny, or do not have the strength, to look at the emotions experienced during the day. If we recognize our experiences, take hold of the situation, respond constructively and meet the challenges, we will immediately understand and express the emotions aroused. Then there will no longer be any need to store their energy in different organs and tissues of the body. The result from our immediate expression of the emotional turmoil of everyday living will of course be that the body is no longer exposed to the same harmful influences. We will experience less pain and other health problems, and thereby access a larger amount of vitality and energy here and now.

Obviously suppressed emotions, incidents and traumas are not the only reasons for the development of symptoms, illnesses and diseases of different kinds. There are many other causes. One reason for deteriorated health is our daily exposure to pollution and chemical substances. The air is filled with poisonous chemical compounds from discharges of many different kinds. The water is "purified" with chlorine. Different metals, nitrogen compounds and bacteria may still be present in the water. In the households and gardens many unhealthy products are handled daily. The crops are sprayed with several different poisons during their short period of growth. They are irrigated with acid rain and "fertilized" with heavy metals from nearby roads and factory complexes. After the harvest the crop is industrially processed to suit our taste. "Processing" of the crops often means that natural vitamins and nutrients are lost and replaced artificially with chemicals. After the processing some food is left deprived of all its vitamins and minerals. The only "enrichment" is the extreme amount of fat that has been added.

One of the most extreme cases in the jungle of processed and maltreated foods is the wholesome potato's way to greasy unhealthy chips deprived of all vitality and nutrition. The food colorants, stabilizers, flavorings, preservatives etc., that are chemically added to the food is not helping in creating a more healthy end product.

Today there is also a risk of unknowingly buying radiated foodstuffs. Radiated products are dead. They completely lack the vital Life Force which is naturally contained in all living matter, and which is so important for the body's and aura's vitality and health. Further, the animals in the meat- and egg-industry are often maltreated. The animals often lead a stressful and undignified life in folds and cages that are far too small for their natural needs. These conditions lead to lower quality of meat and eggs. Many animals are fed growth hormones and antibiotics to keep healthy in their unnatural habitat and to be forced to grow quickly. People take this antibiotic in with their meal, risking resistant bacterial growth in their system, making it far more difficult to treat any disease demanding antibiotics. GMO's (gene modified organisms) might be another health hazard whose effects on the human body are as yet unknown.

How and what we choose to eat also plays an important role in our health. In the stressed society of today it is often difficult to keep regular meal times and create a peaceful family gathering at the table. There are many who do not take the time and effort to cook a well prepared and nutritious meal. It is difficult to find pure foods without residues of heavy metals and other pollutants. Haste and stress in combination with bad eating habits and food stuffs of lesser quality create imbalances in the body and may lead to different kinds of symptoms and diseases.

How regularly we exercise, and our unique genetic constitution also affect the general well-being and health status. Some are born with better odds than others. Some can be delicate and weak or maybe even sick at birth, while others stay sound to the core all through life. The difference is partly due to genetic inheritance. Some people develop asthma, allergies, migraine or ulcers, while others have their weak genes in other parts of the body, therefore being more prone to develop completely different forms of illnesses and symptoms. We are all personalities whose reactions in stressful situations are based on our own references. Some are hardier than others in different situations.

The underlying causes for physical and mental disorders are several. This can lead to difficulties in making the right diagnosis of an illness. Particularly since most diseases spring not from one but several different causes and internal imbalances. For instance, an ulcer might be caused by bad eating habits and irregular meal times during an extended period of time, but it may as well be caused by very hot food, and/or stress at work, worrying about a particular situation, personal problems at work, home or with the family, hereditary disposition, social influence etc., etc. An ulcer can even indicate that one of the thoracic vertebrae connected with the vagus nerve is dislocated. The number of reasons for a physical disorder is infinite, and it is very difficult to diagnose somebody's illness. Nobody without a long medical education has any right to try the art of diagnosis!

The human being consists of a web of energies together forming the intricate energy systems of the body. When applied, the pure, harmonious Reiki energy is automatically attracted to any imbalance in the recipient. Its harmonious energy creates a mirror-image of the imbalanced vibration in the body, all in accordance with the physical law of interference. The two opposing frequencies, Reiki and the disharmonious vibration, simply neutralize each other and harmony is re-created. When the distorted frequencies are harmonized the physical body is strengthened and its natural healing ability is enhanced. This process occurs regardless of the practitioner being aware of the root cause of the problem or not. Reiki is automatically drawn to the areas of energy imbalances. There is absolutely no need for diagnosis, or even any knowledge of anatomy and physiology when treating ourselves or others with Reiki! The entire treatment takes place beyond the little ego. The body is strengthened and the healing process accelerated when the imbalances are harmonized with Reiki. This occurs regardless of where in the body the imbalance originates. Left untreated, energy imbalances may eventually reveal themselves as a physical expression in the body, or they may occur as a psychological imbalance on the emotional or mental level.

Reiki treats with priority, i.e., it is first attracted to the areas of most severe imbalances. Meaning, that the most threatening illnesses and disturbances are attended before the lesser disruptions in the body. It is hence impossible to guide a Reiki treatment. This makes using Reiki a completely ego free activity. The final result of the treatment does not depend on the practitioner but on the Reiki energy radiating from the hands. The recipient automatically draws as much energy as his or her body needs at that particular moment. A large amount of that energy is attracted to the most severe imbalances. Organs and tissues in that area are strengthened and the body's healing curve is sped up to double or more. When the most severe cause for illness has been balanced, the Reiki energy proceeds to work on one problem after the other on a sliding scale of importance.

Both physical and mental disorders are gradually allowed to harmonize through regular Reiki treatments. The time of healing largely depends on how willing the recipient is to let go of the problem or the disease. It is impossible to give a standard table showing the speed of healing for different illnesses and injuries since the underlying causes can vary dramatically. Some individuals are able to see the reason and the underlying meaning of their current disease easier than others. Understanding how badly you have treated yourself and your body will dramatically speed up the healing process, as it is impossible to make necessary changes in life until then. Body constitution and soundness must also be considered. A person with a vital, well exercised body in good condition normally heals faster than someone who has let himself deteriorate to a worn down "couch potato".

Another problem is those individuals who subconsciously have taken on the role of being sick. This act of self-destruction is dramatically affecting their healing process. The illness has become their mission in life. This phenomenon often occurs due to lack of attention and low self worth. Through their illness these people get both attention and care from others. The disease gives them a full-time occupation and an identity.

Unfortunately many people in our society live under such circumstances that their only way of receiving love and affection is to play the role of the sick. This is the dark side of the new mechanistic world, where everybody is expected to be a cog in the machinery without much human contact. Furthermore, as small children we might learn that illness leads to all sorts of "rewards". The child gets to stay home from school and gets mum's whole attention. It gets looked after, stories told, and if it is not too sick it often gets both candy and the favorite food served in bed. Some discover, consciously or subconsciously, how illness can be used as a tool in manipulating others. Reprogramming these conditionings demands time and effort, and a great courage to face one's hidden sides. Reiki can help in this process.

Reiki fills the body with vitality and strength. Disease patterns are balanced and the process of healing is accelerated. Reiki has many exceptional characteristics, but it is an energy science and will not provide magic. In some instances it may seem like a seriously ill body is unaffected by the Reiki energy. The illness has gone too far. Despite regular Reiki treatments there is not enough time for the body to heal itself and the person dies.

At the end of a long and fulfilled life, death is a natural event. But at certain occasions death will seemingly visit too early due to illness, accident or other reasons. In such situations it might be comforting to know that Reiki gives substantial support during the dying process. Terminally ill who are treated with Reiki experience less pain, and the fear of dying is eased. The patient gains in vitality, he seems more alert and can often manage on less or no medical drugs for pain-relief.

Reiki enhances the quality of life, independent of whether we are well or ill, have five days or fifty years left to live, are young or old. Reiki adapts to the existing circumstances creating the harmony, peace and pain-relief that might be needed. Reiki provides extra vitality for each individual, whether healthy, in recovery or dying. Departing from life assisted by Reiki eases the transition and the expected difficulties are fewer. Reiki is the final gift of compassion that we can give to a loved relative or a dear friend.

Reiki works as a valuable complement to all other forms of treatments and therapies. It enhances anything from alternative methods, such as Homeopathy, Acupuncture, Chiropractics, Aroma Therapy, Reflexology, Rolfing, etc., to conventional medicine, which is offering drugs, surgery and other medical treatments. Reiki enhances the positive effect of these therapies and medications. It also reduces any negative influences and side-effects caused by these treatments and drugs. Due to this we see Reiki as a complementary healing technique rather than being simply an alternative.

There are no contra-indications to Reiki. It is never wrong or dangerous to use it. Reiki can be given in combination with drugs and other treatments to strengthen the body, help speed up the healing process, and to give the chosen method of treatment better effect and results. Reiki never disrupts an on-going treatment or medication. In addition, Reiki also enhances the spiritual unfoldment and growth occurring when using techniques such as Meditation, Tai-Chi, Yoga, etc.

Reiki might be the only treatment needed when afflicted by smaller injuries and problems, but it is important not to exclude necessary visits to the doctor. If the least in doubt, see a physician or go to the hospital! Reiki can be given while waiting for the ambulance or the doctor's arrival, or in the car on the way to the hospital. To give Reiki as soon as possible after a severe accident can, and has, saved lives. This does of course not mean that you should exclude necessary medical treatments! At the scene of an accident, or if somebody falls dramatically ill, urgent medical treatment is often necessary. But in this context Reiki has sometimes become the link between life and death while waiting for the ambulance to arrive or the injured person to reach the hospital.

SUMMARY
- Reiki requires no diagnosis.
- Reiki treats with priority.

- Reiki is an extraordinary complement to all other treatments, therapies and medications.
- Reiki has no contra-indications.
- Reiki is totally safe, has no side-effects, and can never be overdosed.
- Reiki provides an outstanding stress-release and relaxation.

Reiki maximizes your health potential on all levels. Reiki is an irreplaceable first-aid kit always at hand. But the most important characteristic of Reiki is its preventive effect. Strength, energy and vitality are maximized in the body when Reiki is applied on a regular basis. Furthermore, many imbalances are harmonized even before manifesting as symptoms in the body. Many unnecessary problems and diseases are thereby avoided on all levels: physically, emotionally, mentally and spiritually.

FIVE

BEYOND THE PHYSICAL

*H*uman beings are not able to consciously utilize more than about ten percent of the brain's capacity. Many researchers claim we do not use more than two or three, maybe up to seven or eight percent of the brain actively. I usually say ten percent when speaking of what is hidden beyond the body, in the meandering space of the brain. Ten percent is still a very low conscious utilization of the body's most fine-tuned organ.

The part of the brain actively in use is called the conscious mind, or ego. This faculty takes care of all thinking, logic, reasoning and intellect. The remaining approximately ninety percent of the brain contains the subconscious mind, i.e., all the memories, experiences, previous conditioning, belief systems and instinct, as well as the superconscious mind where higher spiritual values, intuition and conscience originate.

The subconscious mind, sometimes called the lower self or inner child, expresses the basic needs of survival. Here are all the hidden gifts, talents and fundamental drives. The spontaneous reactions of the subconscious mind can be compared to the reactions of a four-to-six year old child. And just like a small child it is also very open to different kinds of suggestions and influences. The subconscious mind can therefore be of good help when trying to positively change some part of the personality or heal the body through affirmations, hypnosis and visualization.

Unfortunately, it is much more common that the subconscious mind is programmed to work in the opposite direction. We tend to continuously repeat negative statements about ourselves and others by perpetually pointing out apparent and hidden imperfections and defects. The lower self is as susceptible to negative influences as to positive. When rambling on about our drawbacks we therefore thoughtlessly build up negative opinions and beliefs about ourselves. On top of this the logical and reasoning ego often takes over, rationalizing the inner child's instinctive feelings and premonitions, just like a parent often reproves and underestimates the feelings and needs of a small child. That way the inner child's natural spontaneity, inspiration and playfulness may be suppressed. We might lose contact with our feelings and instinct, since the inner child has a tendency to withdraw to escape the attacks of the ego. This can eventually lead to blocked energies in the body, lowered immune defense and a tendency for self-destruction in the things we do.

The superconscious mind is sometimes called the higher self. Its function is to remind the ego about the spiritual opportunities that exist beyond the materialistic world and the limitations of the conscious mind (the ego). All universal knowledge is stored within the higher self. At times we might be able to intuitively tap into the insights originating from this pool of knowledge even though we often lack a conscious link with it. The poor communication with the higher self is due to imbalances between the ego and the lower self. We lose contact with the superconscious mind when we get stuck in the tug-of-war between the logic of the ego and the instincts, needs and feelings of the lower self.

Soul, a spark of Light and our true essence, is also located deep within. Soul is the embodiment of all we are and have ever been. It is immortal, and continuously developing through our human experiences. Soul communicates with the ego via the higher self. Our task is to recreate the balance between the lower self and the ego, to make it possible to reinstate the lost connection between the ego and the higher self. Only in achieving inner balance is it possible to open the door to the abundance of the enduring wisdom within the higher self, where the solutions to all problems and answers to all questions dwell.

We can release blocked energy and experience a freer body, improved health, greater joy, increased spontaneity, courage, wisdom and understanding, by becoming more aware of the relationship between the ego and the higher and lower selves. In this chapter you can read about how the human being grows into her own personality through her experiences in life. The internal role-plays and disagreements taking place between the subconscious and the conscious minds are reflected in our external lives, in the roles we choose to play out here.

OPENING THE COMMUNICATION WITH THE HIGHER SELF

In all possible ways the conscious mind (the ego) tries to contact the forgotten higher aspects within. New-born babies still remember they are Soul. They are completely open and have total communication with the Spiritual Worlds. Unfortunately this interaction is gradually closed down as they grow and develop into adult human beings. The cutting off from Soul and the distancing from the Inner Worlds often leads to various states of sadness, depression, aggression and frustration, or feelings of disorientation, alienation, loneliness and inner yearning.

More or less consciously, every person is trying to reestablish the lost contact with the higher self and Soul. The unconscious search often manifests in excessive use of various drugs such as alcohol, narcotics, etc. Smoking, over eating, and excessive sexual interactions are also expressions of the lower self's need to fill the inner hollow by external means.

A more conscious search might be carried out by joining various teachings, traditions or schools. This may include all kinds of activities, such as looking into the different activities offered within the Human Potential field and the New-Age movement, or attending various types of churches, religions, spiritual paths and cults. Other alternatives include searching in books, or participating in various seminars. This type of conscious search often helps to find answers that lead to a deeper understanding of the totality. Joining a community, a movement or a church has sometimes offered exactly the support a certain person needed in order to continue his unfoldment. To other people the external knowledge offered from different groups leaves many questions unanswered. The inner feeling of emptiness remains untouched. Reading this book probably means that you already have experienced this persistent urge to find the hidden answers to your secret quest. You sense that life contains more, a something that you cannot yet give a name. Perhaps you have searched in vain in books, seminars and religions, or maybe you have visited psychics, channelers, clairvoyants or gurus of various kinds, but you are still experiencing that you are yet to find the answer to how to fill that inner void and reduce the coldness within.

Reiki offers an invaluable technique in helping to re-establish the communication between the ego and the higher self. Finding true freedom of Soul, and to fully reconnect with Its wisdom would take many lifetimes of dedicated effort and consecration. It is not achievable in one lifetime. With the help of various techniques and active effort however, it might be possible to gradually develop an inner communication and understanding. The attunements of the First Reiki Degree expands the awareness, and establishes a stronger communication between outer and inner dimensions. Reiki assists in utilizing the capacity of the brain more consciously. We achieve greater harmony and an increased ability to listen within for the wisdom of the higher self and Soul. In addition we develop inner strength, increased capacity to love, and ability to replace our feelings of lack and emptiness with compassion, warmth and confidence.

There are no obligations or belief system connected to Reiki, and we do not become members of any association or movement when participating in a Reiki seminar. No follow-up is required, and all contact with the Reiki instructor can be relinquished after the end of the seminar.

Once the energy has been activated Reiki remains in the body for the rest of one's life, regardless of whether contact with the Reiki Master is maintained or not. Reiki helps us take responsibility, and to understand that we and nobody else, are the ones to fulfill our own lives.

RESPONSIBILITY

It may be uncomfortable to hear, but it is really only you who can decide how you feel. No other person has the ability to change your state of mind unless you agree to it on some level. It might be difficult to grasp this concept, since at an early age we abdicate the responsibility for ourselves and our situation to others. We quickly learn that our parents take control and make decisions for us when we are small. Teachers take over some of the responsibility for education and development when we start school. We grow into adulthood, but unfortunately often forget to reclaim the responsibility we once gave away as children. Instead we expect others to change our lives for us. We accuse family members, friends, work colleagues, bosses, doctors, lawyers, politicians and others of having created the situations we face, and for being the reason to why we do not feel well and happy. We have simply forgotten that on some level we have created all the events that are coming into our life.

It is you and nobody else who decides how you will feel and react in a certain situation. Happiness or unhappiness are just different expressions of your emotional stage. No one outside of yourself can create the emotions you hold within. That would be impossible. Other people and events can push your buttons. They can act as catalysts in a chain of events that eventually lead you to explode in anger, fear, tears, sadness or with any other emotion that you hold. However, those emotions do not come from anybody else. They come from within yourself. It is you who create the emotions that you feel.

Everything that we have ever experienced, from early childhood until today, has contributed to our own particular view on life. Through our experiences we develop into unique individuals. Each person will therefore react in a unique way to the situations that he or she faces. What upsets one person may not be perceived as a drama by another. Previous conditioning and influences lead to expectations, belief systems and opinions about ourselves and others. We create different attitudes to life and to our everyday experiences. These previous experiences influence our reactions in future events. We often believe that other people are treating us badly, when in reality it is we who decide to feel badly treated. We have developed an idea of how we want to be treated, and if that does not happen we feel wronged and become angry or sad, or experience other emotional reactions. We allow others to decide how we feel by letting them make us upset. The fault however, is nobody else's but our own.

Human beings carry loads of unresolved conflicts, traumas and expectations that lead to various reactions when interacting with others. In order to learn how to respond rather than having out of control reactions, it is important that we reclaim responsibility for ourselves and our situation. Foremost by admitting the fact that we have complete control over our own lives and actions. That we have absolute responsibility! The next step is to resume the contact with our inner selves, where all the conditioning and belief systems have their foundation. By using Reiki on a regular basis we receive an effective tool in communicating with our inner selves, and to see and understand the patterns that tend to repeat themselves in our lives. Only then is it possible to change our way of behavior. Once we become aware of our previous conditioning we can consciously choose to change and let go. The decision to make that change is possible to take at any time in life. You are never too old or too young to decide to change your attitude to life, and thereby causing a positive changing in your personality.

NEGATIVE INFLUENCE

Previous experiences and memories are mainly stored in the large inactive part of the brain which we have little or no conscious contact with. Everything we have been trained to think about ourselves is stored there. In each person's interior, there are many different opinions and values about oneself and society, and they are all related to upbringing and previous experiences. Many people have a subconscious mind filled with negative opinions and ideas about how bad and useless they are. The subconscious mind fools us into believing that we are not as good as others and that we are not worthy of a good, happy and comfortable life. On a conscious level, we know very well what we want and need and we try in every possible way to reach contentment in life. We strive for a well-paid and stimulating job, a new fancy car, a beautiful cozy home, a well-adjusted family, an exciting spare time, a loving and trusting relationship with a perfect partner, etc. Despite all efforts to create a perfect life, we will have difficulties in finding happiness as long as the subconscious mind, due to previous influences and beliefs of what we really deserve, works in the opposite direction. It does not matter how much we want something. Conditioning will always over rule the conscious will as it is deeply manifested in the unconscious mind which is ninety percent of the brain. To fulfill our desires we first have to change our ingrown beliefs and attitudes.

In growing into adults we go through different stages. A new born baby lives a joyful life, literally being the center of the universe, the whole world revolving around its own self. All its needs are taken care of, be it food, warmth, contact, love or dry diapers. The child knows it is a perfect being. From this stage of inner contentment the child moves into the stage of influence. The personality is developing, based on parents' and other's opinions, behavior and programming. Society, culture and religion also have a strong influence. The child starts to become aware of its surroundings and its own limitations.

The brain in a newborn baby is not yet fully developed, but it evolves quickly the first few years through experiences and stimulation from the environment. All the new experiences in a baby's life causes millions of new nerve synapses to form in the brain. This evolution refines the brain's work of cataloguing information and drawing conclusions, and it is enhancing the ability to see connections and to understand. This process continues throughout life, but is most evident during the first few years when the intellect is rapidly developing.

Each time a child is criticized a nerve synapse with a negative charge that will lead to further insecurity and low self-esteem is formed in the brain. Adults too, may find themselves in situations where they are criticized. The synapses formed in their childhood are then further reinforced. The message to the brain is: "You are a failure!". When young we often get this message, together with other harmful statements such as: "You can't...", "You are not able to...", "You don't understand...", etc. This negative programming is nothing but verbal abuse, and forms the foundation to the belief that we are not good enough as we are. We start comparing ourselves with others. In that comparison we always seem to be the loser. We constantly seem to find others who have greater capabilities, more intelligence, and better physical appearance than ourselves. In comparing, we make ourselves believe in lack and inferiority. We start to feel unsuccessful, and begin to develop low self-worth and various complexes.

The personality is developing this way. The more negative experiences we have during our childhood and while growing up, the more we learn to disapprove of ourselves, and the lower the self-worth as adults. The more support and approval, the more unconditional love and acceptance, and the more trust we are given when little, the stronger and more secure we become as adults.

MASKS, ARMOR AND ROLES

Our personality is gradually developing from the images we create of ourselves. To protect our vulnerable, and as we might believe unacceptable self, we build invisible walls and armor. Later nobody is allowed inside this armor in our fear of being hurt. We live with a distorted image of who we think we are, and how we think we should be in order to be accepted and loved by others. We start behaving in ways we think other people want or expect us to behave. We hide behind armor and masks and play altered roles in different situations. All of this to protect ourselves from other people realizing who we really are.

The human being is a group animal, and his ancient instinct tells him that belonging to the flock is his only chance of survival. Even today, the worst thing that can happen to a person is being excluded from the "tribe" he feels he belongs to. It is immensely important to man to fit into the group he has chosen. To most people this group is represented by country, culture, society, and on a minor scale, different social groups. Hence, we form ourselves according to both unspoken rules and written laws. To be sure to fit in, we put on various masks and act out different roles. The exterior facade these role-games and masks present is interpreted by others as our personality.

The masks that hide our inner can include anything from make-up and clothes to various titles, etc. Most people choose to dress within the limits established by culture and fashion not to attract too much attention. To the best of our ability, we try to avoid being conspicuous and different. We play the role of being "just right". We push our True Self and suppressed needs aside, and hide behind just the right clothes, just the right make-up and just the right titles we have procured through work and other activities. Nobody knows any longer who we really are, what we feel and how we see ourselves and our lives.

Some people are outside the scope of society and no longer follow the established rules and laws. These people have just as big a need of belonging to a group, and are equally as stuck in the system as everybody else. The difference is that they adopt other rules, and dress and behave in another way than what is commonly accepted in society. They often have a common interest, for example protesting against society and the establishment. These groups can represent anything from hippies to skinheads or any other gang or cult. Despite their rebellious tendencies, they are very careful to follow the rules established by their own group, regarding clothes, behavior and opinions. Their rules and unwritten laws may be totally different from those of the society, but must nevertheless be followed by the members in order for them to be allowed in the group.

We unconsciously accept the roles we play and the masks we wear to protect ourselves. We are totally unaware of being absorbed by these roles and beliefs about ourselves and others, until one day we consciously decide to observe ourselves and our relationship with the environment. Many times we play our roles so well that we forget who we really are, and thus completely lose touch with our true inner selves. That is when the emptiness inside becomes too painful. We feel isolated, and the loneliness and inner yearning can be difficult to handle. We no longer know who we really are and the pain caused in disowning our true inner core can be excruciating. The agony becomes especially difficult if we are consciously unaware of its origin.

MANIPULATION

Other people form an opinion about who we are by the roles we play and the exterior image we present of ourselves. We can appear strong and confident or weak and helpless. Many times we try to manipulate those around us with our games. This can be done both consciously and unconsciously. Manipulation can have its roots as far back as childhood. For instance, by observing our parents' relationship, we might skillfully learn how to get things our way. Many people are excellent manipulators. By acting in certain ways they make other people give them more attention and more advantages. By acting feeble and incapable, they get more help and support from others. By being weak and ill, they receive more attention and care. By riding on somebody's sense of guilt, they buy advantages, and by threat and intimidation they conquer other people's will. They are simply trying to buy love by using calculating and devious methods.

Most of these psychological role-games take place beyond the conscious mind. They are played out deep inside our being, where they are based on previous conditioning and belief systems. Manipulation is often such an integrated part of the self that we seldom notice when we play people out against each other to gain advantages. Nobody is completely free from the tendency to manipulate, but in some this characteristic is more dominant then in others. We weaken ourselves when manipulating and controlling, but there is no opening to change until we consciously start looking at ourselves and our tactics. To use and to be used confines us in a dependency that is easier to break out of once we become aware of the games we are playing.

CHANGE

Many people walk through life without ever understanding how little is needed to change the situation they live in. They will continue leading an unsatisfactory life as long as they cannot accept who they are. They create an illusion of themselves because they are afraid of what is hiding inside. The perfect being dwelling within has been

pushed aside and forgotten. Instead we focus on all that is wrong in
life and on everybody that we think is doing us injustice. We criticize
and judge excessively without understanding that every word of
blame is an indirect attack on ourselves. If we understood the whole
world is a mirror of ourselves and that all the people we meet are our
teachers, we would soon treat both ourselves and others differently.

The first step is to look at life with a new and more open attitude. The School of Life constantly offers experiences, events and
situations that help us unfold. Each change we go through is yet
another step ahead in our growth. The people we meet on our way
through life help us look at ourselves with new eyes, and to discover
parts in our personality that we might need to change. If we are having problems to cooperate with, or accepting a particular person, we
can be quite sure he or she reflects a suppressed part of ourselves. We
unconsciously hide characteristics that we do not like in ourselves, and
when we see them in others we are quick to criticize and judge. That
which we have suppressed leaves a vacuum that invariably attracts
more of the same to create a balance. Due to this we will constantly
attract people who openly show the attributes that we have hidden.
We will continue to do this until we realize how these seemingly obnox-
ious people reflect our own internal blockages. When we have learned
this lesson we can start altering our attitude by observing these people, and hence proceed to change our own way of behavior. Instead
of letting some people ruin our life, we can perceive them as the
teachers and masters they really are. Once we are able to do that, we
will be more capable of grasping that these people are not just generally unpleasant and hopeless to deal with. They also have the kindness
to show us what we need to work on in our own personality. If
allowed to, these people can provide us with a new awareness of our
internal affairs.

To be able to grow into fulfillment and balance, we must first dare
to look at ourselves, and the habits and reaction patterns we have developed. This can be difficult since we to a large extent are ruled by the
subconscious mind where these conditions and believes are harbored.
The contact with our True Self is often totally or partly severed. We

are therefore quite unaware of how we play the game of life and the limiting effects of an unbalanced inner. We are so involved in ourselves that it is difficult to see our own shortcomings and the role-plays we are constantly participating in.

FREEDOM OF CHOICE

If we give away the responsibility for how we feel to others, we fall victim to circumstances and are helplessly held in the present situation. We lose control and think that everybody except ourselves rules emotions, events and situations in our life. When stuck in a situation like that it can feel very real, but this is just an illusion created because we have given it permission to appear. We have simply forgotten the inherited ability to create our own reality. Nothing will be different until you start acting, and taking responsibility for the changes you want to manifest. You will achieve nothing by accusing others for the events coming into your life. Every emotion, experience and situation is created by yourself. Everything you see and experience are products of your own mind. This of course, also means that you have complete control over everything that happens around you. By accepting active responsibility for your present situation your inner strength is increased and you will grow as a human being.

All the choices you have made and all the decisions you have once taken, everything from the education you selected to the people you choose to share your life with, have created your present situation. At every new crossroads, and at every new opportunity, you have the chance to change your future. The education you chose has given you the career opportunities you now have. The place you live in today gives you few or many opportunities to expand. The people you have chosen to have around you, help you develop in a certain direction. They enhance or hold you back in your growth process. Even the minor choices you make every day assist in creating your future. For example how you choose to react in a particular situation, what you choose to do in your spare time, the furniture you select for your house and even what you choose to have for dinner. In conclusion: everything you have ever done up till today, and all the decisions you have previously made, have brought you to your present position and have given you everything you have today. If you are not content with what you have or with yourself you can choose to change at any moment. Everything you do today decides what your tomorrow will be. If you look at life with negative eyes, you will meet the darkness you have already anticipated. If you have a positive and joyful outlook on life, you will create a fulfilled and happy future for yourself.

If it seems impossible to change your situation there is always the possibility of changing your attitude. You invariably have the freedom to choose how to react or respond in each situation you are confronted with. If you are unhappy in your present situation but do not have the ability or strength to change, it is very important that you change your *attitude* to whatever it is that is tormenting you. For example, you might not dare to resign from your present job in fear of not finding another. If you choose to remain in a situation like that it is vital that you change your attitude towards the work you do, your work mates, or whatever other things that are bothering you. If you do not, the risk of developing bodily symptoms and problems by time is increased many fold. You can become ill from staying in a situation where you are distressed, unless you change your attitude to the problem. Illness is the body's own way of showing imbalances in your life situation. You can learn to look at your life with different eyes and with greater joy and appreciation. If you change your attitude, your feelings towards the problems will change or lessen, and you will feel better and experience less stress in life.

Sometimes the lesson in the situation may be as simple as just *accepting* what you have, or the particularly "annoying" people you have around you. In our growth process we must learn to accept that other people view life differently from us. Each and every one has a unique image of the world based on earlier references and experiences. This means that we see and meet things in different ways. Imagine, for example, that five of six people are watching a particular movie. They all watch the same movie, but when they recite the film to the sixth person they will give different versions of what happened. Each one has focused on the parts of the movie that is important to him or her. The sixth person listening to the five stories finally thinks he is given the story of five different movies. This is because the five people who saw the movie have different backgrounds and frames of reference, they each reacted individually to the story, and different parts were important to each one.

Life works the same way. We are all actors and directors in the same film, but because of different experiences we interpret the events in our life-movie in different ways. Each and every one has their own truth and unique image of life and how it should be lived. Therefore, we cannot claim that our opinion is the only valid one. Every individual lives his own truth, and many times that truth can be completely different from other peoples ideas and convictions. Therefore, we have no right to make judgments about other peoples view on life or the way they live. For them, the image of the world they have created is the only truth they understand. You cannot change that by claiming your truth is better or more genuine than theirs.

If you think that someone behaves wrongly or in a foolish manner, it is because that person has a totally different viewpoint of what is going on compared to you. He or she acts in the way deemed most appropriate according to his or her experiences and understanding. Maybe this clashes with what you think is right, but you still have no right to interfere in these people's lives. You must give them the same freedom to lead their own lives as you expect them to give you to lead yours. If you try to interfere and to run other people's lives, regardless of how right you think you are and how wrongly you think they act, you too will meet people who will try to influence and interfere with the life that you lead. If you radiate trust and understanding of other people's characteristics, you will be met by warmth and openness. If you give others the freedom to live their truth, you will meet the same freedom to lead the life you have chosen. If you force yourself on other people, interfering with their lives, your own life in turn will be locked and limited by opinions and attitudes forced on to you by others.

All the experiences you are given come to you for particular reasons, and everything that happens to you has a perfect cause. Life is a school, and our daily experiences give us opportunities to learn more in particular areas of need. There is no such thing as a wrong decision since the choices we make shows that we need more understanding and experience in that particular area of life. Sometimes we might face choices that seem almost impossible to make. We are forced to choose between "the rock and the hard place" and no matter what we do, the final result is not going to be anything we would have wished for. Why then accuse yourself in retrospect? You did your very best under the circumstances. We waste too much valuable time regretting yesterday rather than getting on with the life we live today. We lose far too much vital energy by living in yesterday's memories, accusing ourselves and others for the life these previous events have given us today. Reclaiming control of our present situation gives more energy and increased vitality here and now.

The Tide of Life

Life consists of a string of "ups" and "downs". There are moments of joy and times of sorrow, troublesome and easy events and situations in a never ending blend. All these highs and lows we encounter *are* life! Nobody is spared distressing experiences. It is through the difficult times in life we grow and unfold. Each time we manage through a particularly difficult time we gain renewed strength. We have grown with the situation and developed greater wisdom on the way. Through grief we are polished, learning patience and compassion towards others. The time of suffering presents an opportunity to develop courage, strength and understanding, but it is only you who can make the decision to evolve beyond the difficult situation. At times it might seem as if the easiest solution is to hang on to the darkness, staying in the bitterness and victim consciousness. During these times of hurt, do not forget that everyone has to meet difficulties in life. Maybe someone's trouble seems small and insignificant compared to somebody else's exposed and difficult life, but everybody gets allotted as much as they can handle. Even the seemingly small events can be experienced very strongly by the person affected. We cannot judge somebody else for their reactions, but we can develop understanding and love for people in pain by dealing with our own difficult experiences. When we have managed through a difficult period, we often undergo a time of calm and harmony.

Life is not about never losing control. To walk the razors edge of life is not an easy balancing act. Life is rather a question of how quickly we choose to rise once we have lost our equilibrium. The knocks of life can be hard and at times it is easy to fall. Someone might choose to stay in the pit of sorrow and self-pity for months and years, or maybe a whole life, while others quickly rise to take the next round. It does not matter how much help you are given from family, friends, acquaintances, therapists or counselors, you will not move on until *you* take an active decision to start feeling better. I am not saying that you should hide and suppress grief and other emotions, since that will damage your body severely. But I do say that you can *choose* happiness over sorrow, and love over anger and hatred. Accept that which has happened, and that this is how your situation is at the moment.

It is actually possible to feel the stir of inherent joy even in the middle of the deepest grief and pain. The joy that dwells within comes from your True Self. Soul is always happy, independent of the circumstances you find yourself in. It is always possible to contact the true joy flowing from Soul and to draw on Its strength. To be able to do so it might first be necessary to throw out old baggage from previous experiences and influences. These are conditionings holding you back and limiting your understanding of the universal connection which exists between the ego and the higher divine aspects.

Reiki expands the awareness and makes it easier to see the belief systems and conditionings that have ruled life until today. By using Reiki regularly, we see and understand more of the patterns that keep repeating themselves in our lives. We gain strength to actively change opinions and ideas and thereby releasing the blocked energy that previous beliefs have locked inside us. Consistent use of Reiki makes us more aware of the relationship with our surroundings, and how we try to satisfy our internal needs with external factors. Increased awareness is the same as increased knowledge and understanding. In other words, Reiki creates a more open communication with the higher self and forms an increased access to the collective universal knowledge. It becomes easier to listen within when we are more aware. We realize that all answers and solutions can be found inside ourselves. Self worth is strengthened. We develop control and independence in a positive spiral of growth and insight.

THE OBSERVER WITHIN

You can actively help your growth process along by developing an independent observer within. This is a small part of yourself, able to look at the situation with totally objective eyes. The internal observer is not critical or judgmental in any way. It does not attack what you or others are doing or telling you how foolishly you or they behave. If you would hear such a voice rising from inside, be sure that it is your partial and prejudiced lower self that is talking. The Observer within observes without judgment. It objectively takes in the whole situation and the opinions of everyone involved. It gathers all the facts without being fixed on a particular end result. The Observer sees events objectively, and makes you aware of patterns and situations that are repeated time and time again. It makes it easier to see what could have been done differently to obtain another outcome. It helps you see things the way they really are, and acts as a catalyst in an effective cleansing process. You can rid yourself of much unnecessary baggage by trying to constantly be aware of how you act or react in the daily situations facing you.

DETACHMENT

It is easier not to react out of balance and in an uncontrolled way if you consciously work on your behavior with the help of the inner Observer. You will then become more detached to others' reactions and opinions. Evolving is an art. People who develop with most ease practice detachment, one of the most important traits of the personality. Detachment does *not* mean developing coldness, insensitivity, calculation, distancing or isolation. Detachment is about the deep inner knowing that you have complete responsibility for your own self. This is developing from the knowledge that true happiness can only come from within. A person that has developed detachment knows that everything he needs in life emerges from his own inner.

Attachment is the opposite to detachment and acts as a severe limitation to our growth process. Being attached to people, things and results is a constant source of discomfort and pain. In losing that which we are emotionally attached to we are thrown into a personal disaster or crisis. We might lose control totally. Whatever it is that we are emotionally attached to has now taken control of our life! We allow ourselves to become victims of circumstances, and as a consequence we experience negative emotional turmoil and pain.

If you stay detached you know that absolutely nothing in life can affect your inner joy. If you lose something, you try to see what can be learned from the situation. You dare to live your life with passion and spontaneity since you are not afraid of losing what you presently have around you. You allow yourself to live totally and fully. You know that nothing in life is static, that both people, things and situations come and go. But if you are attached to what you have gathered around you, you will constantly be torn between who you really are and how you think you must act, to be able to keep what you call yours. You restrain yourself and your spontaneity in fear of what others might think about what you do and who you are. By different activities you try to keep a situation static because you are afraid that change will lead to loss. Detachment on the other hand is a way of being. It lessens the burden of worry and creates greater freedom to live. After detaching from the fear of loss you dare embrace life with joy and passion, and without inhibitions.

If you dare to express your True Self openly, others will treat you with new respect. They will be attracted by the strength you radiate, and lifted by the joy that is reflecting from your inner. In this way you can help to change the world. Your greatest ability to make this change real is simply by changing yourself. It is not possible to create a different world if you choose to hold on to your own state of stagnation. Those around you are affected by your development. They are lifted by your openness and joy, and can in their turn spread the joy you have aroused in them to others. In this way, openness and joy are spread amongst people like rings on the water. You can never change somebody else in any other way than by changing yourself. If all people chose to change themselves, rather than complaining about other peoples' faults and shortcomings, hatred, misery, starvation and war would dry up due to lack of negative nourishment. Therefore, let go of anger, criticism and judgment. Open yourself to joy and compassion and you too can spread rings of love over the waters of earth, contributing to a positive change!

You will lead a more accomplished life if you develop detachment, since you no longer are expecting particular results. Expectations often cause disappointments because you tie yourself to results that most often will never be realized. For instance, there are more suicides committed on Christmas Day than on any other day of the year due to shattered expectations and broken illusions. For the same reasons we have an enormous peak in the divorce rate after the summer holidays. For almost a year we are looking forward to a few weeks of free time when we expect everything to be perfect and just the way we imagined. Reality often turns out completely different. Unrealistic expectations put on the present situation lead to dissatisfaction, and it is easy to accuse others of causing our own disappointment. If you are not attached to how the weekend, the holiday or something else you have planned will turn out, you will give these events a chance to develop in an uninterrupted and harmonious way. Whatever happens will be perfect since you have not placed any limiting expectations on the outcome.

RELATIONSHIPS

To a greater or lesser degree everyone is harboring unresolved inner imbalances and blockages. For instance, we often have great difficulties in expressing our internal masculine and feminine energies in a balanced way. Instead we are inclined to use our dominant side, where women tend to primarily use their feminine qualities while men primarily use their masculine characteristics. These roles can of course be reversed, where the woman expresses strong masculine characteristics while the man is perceived as weak and feminine. Unconsciously we are trying to find a partner who is able to mirror our suppressed Yin/Yang characteristics. This is called projection, and it makes it difficult to develop fully harmonious relationships with others. The more intimate the relationship, the more obvious the reflection of our own needs put on to the other person. We expect him or her to give us what we lack. We demand that he or she changes so that we will be able to express ourselves more perfectly. We thereby place the responsibility for our inability to realize certain characteristics inside of ourselves on to somebody else. Another person's behavior and attitude is of course important in a relationship, but our strength lies in realizing our right to change ourselves. At any moment we can start giving of ourselves, instead of constantly and at all costs seek satisfaction and self gratification in our relationship with others.

The choice of partner in a relationship always reflects your own state of mind. If your partner does not treat you with respect and consideration, it is probably because you treat yourself with depreciation. If your partner criticizes you, it is because he or she reflects your own self-criticism and perfectionism. If you feel unloved and neglected, it is because of your own self-hatred and lack of appreciation. A person with internal imbalances is in a sense incomplete. He or she will therefore always attract other incomplete people. Incomplete people also have a tendency to be dissatisfied with each other because each reflects what the other one lacks. This pattern will be repeated until you can see your own shortcomings and choose to do something about them. It serves no purpose to try to change the other person. You must change yourself in order for the results to be real and lasting.

Not until you accept yourself as you are, realize your own worth, and harmoniously express your feminine and masculine qualities, will you be able to attract other balanced people. Then you will attract somebody who vibrates in the same energy as you, and it will be easier to build a relationship based on acceptance and unconditional love since you project fewer characteristics and expectations on each other. Which ever state you find yourself in, relationships offer invaluable opportunities for development and growth.

LOVE
     As long as we use others to correct our own imperfections, we will also be ridden by a strong urge to change the imperfections shown to us by these people. Since we have suppressed these shortcomings in ourselves we perceive them as faults when seen in others. In a rela-

tionship we then tie ourselves together by demands, expectations and the need to correct the other person's flaws. The pressure and tension in the relationship is increased when it becomes evident that we cannot fill each other's endless needs. The fear of losing the other and of not being good enough is increased, and the demands on one another are constantly elevating. The result is a stressed and loveless relationship based on anticipations such as: "I love you if you..." and "If you really loved me you would....". These expectations have absolutely nothing to do with true love. Love is completely free of demands, and totally accepting in itself. Love leaves space and freedom for individual growth. It gives without expecting anything in return. True love is unconditional and completely liberated from the need to perform.

Our true task in life is to develop and give unconditional love. That is why we associate with others and go through various relationships. Both intimate and superficial relationships help us see ourselves as who we are, and to study the patterns that have a tendency to repeat themselves in life. We are given a new opportunity to change and to approach the situation from a different angle with each new encounter. Every attempt leads to further development and understanding. In time we can see where we previously went wrong and what we can do to change future outcomes.

We learn lessons in all our relationships. First we try to change and improve everybody and everything except ourselves, until one day we might see the bigger picture. Our own change can only begin when we become aware of these games. When we realize that we can never escape ourselves by changing the external situation, change partners, hide behind work, or any other made up reason. The great change will occur when you accept and love yourself just the way you are, when you realize your own worth and start to appreciate and respect yourself fully.

To love and accept oneself has nothing to do with conceit or being selfish. A conceited person has a low self-esteem that he is trying to boost by asserting himself, constantly showing off his advantages.

It is easy to see through such a person. He uses different tricks when trying to outshine others, and gain for himself at other's expense. The need for other people's praise and appreciation is perpetual, since the conceit is only a false facade that hides loneliness, insecurity and self-contempt. A person who accepts and respects himself on the other hand has no need to shine in front of others. By loving himself he can love others and enjoy giving without demands and expectations of his own. He has developed an inner strength and security, and has no need to look for reassurance from others. Such a person knows that all human beings are perfect creatures, and that he is a part of a greater wholeness.

SURRENDER

As a natural part of our development we let go of people who no longer have the ability to follow our vision. Every individual has their own goals, conceptions and life plan. It is not unusual that we develop in different directions from the people around us. That is part of the dynamics of life. We reach crossings where the roads fork, we thank each other for the learning experiences we have shared, and depart in happiness and love. It is important to learn to distinguish between the separations that are a natural part of our development, and the disconnections occurring as a result of our internal imbalances and external mirroring. If you can let go of a person or situation with love and compassion it is probably time to move on, but if you feel rage, hatred, regrets, insecurity, criticism or other indignant emotions you probably have more to learn from the situation. Our ability to interpret different situations, and to understand that the decisions we make spring from either harmonious love or uncontrollable emotional turmoil, grows with increased self-awareness.

Daily events help us see where we need to change, and what it is we must surrender to be able to move on. Some incidents occur in order to help us develop greater understanding and love for ourselves and others. Some obstacles arise to teach us how to accept. If you are able to totally accept a situation or an event in your life, despite that it is not to your advantage, then you have really surrendered. When you accept a situation exactly as it is, you open the door to change, and make it possible for the situation to take on a new direction. In this process you learn trust and unconditional love. Furthermore, your life becomes so much easier when you do not constantly have to fight to get your own ideas and demands met. Instead you surrender your little self to trustingly go with the universal flow of wisdom and perfection.

Of course you actively take care of yourself and your problems, but there will always be a time when you have to surrender. When you have done your very best and there is nothing more to do, letting go of the anxiety around the problem or situation is the next vital step to take. To be able to find a solution to your problem you first have to let go of any expectations of the outcome. If you expect a particular result, you automatically exclude many of the opportunities that may offer themselves along the way because they seemingly do not fit into your own fixed solution. You deny yourself of many new experiences this way, and life becomes harder than necessary.

The door to future opportunities and fortunes opens inwardly. If you stubbornly bang your head against the door vainly trying to open it, you will only get a headache. If you instead step back, surrendering the situation, the door will easily swing open. In lifting your head when stepping back, you will be able to see all the other doors that are already wide open in waiting. There are endless opportunities behind each and every one of these doors. If you continue to strive in vain towards the only solution you are able see with your limited understanding, you will miss all these new chances and opportunities. As long as you persist in holding on to the situation through anxiety or awkward attempts to do things your way, the natural flow is obstructed and the problem remains.

It is not only problems, things and situations we sometimes need to surrender, it could also be people. Love is impossible to control. The more we try to hold onto somebody else, the more forceful the reaction will be. We own nobody and nothing. A person who believes that other living beings can be tied down and kept by threats has not understood that love is free. The need of forcing oneself upon others derives from insecurity and low self-worth. If you free yourself and detach from external factors, people and belongings, you will start to vibrate harmonious energy. This harmony will attract enjoyable and positive events, and your life will become rich and filled with true love.

LIVING SPIRITUALLY

It is not always easy to live in a state of balance. Life constantly gives us new opportunities to grow and develop by providing us with all kinds of challenges. Sometimes it is possible to keep a good mood, at other times we explode in a blustering emotional outburst. It is obviously natural not to be able to meet adversity with happy smiles at all times. Contentment and love is what we are here to learn.

For myself, in trying to maintain my inner balance, I keep certain key words in mind. They are especially helpful when life is difficult. These memory keys were born one day when I was pondering about how to most easily express the philosophy of life that I had arrived at. The basic principles of living a more spiritual life are gathered in these six short paragraphs:

AWARENESS: Be aware of who you are and your purpose in life. That you have total responsibility for everything you create around you. Be aware that you are Soul, a spark of God, and therefore indestructible! Hold your awareness of the other key words: detachment, unconditional love, responsibility, surrender and gratitude, and try to live by them.

DETACHMENT: Be detached to people, things and events, and to the final outcome and solution to situations and problems. Do not expect particular results. Be an uncritical observer to your own actions. Do not react. Do not judge. Simply observe how you act in different situations and learn from it. If you think that something could have been done in another way, tell yourself that: "next time I will do it differently".

UNCONDITIONAL LOVE: Love without conditions. Total acceptance of yourself and others, precisely as you and they are. Unconditional love is love without strings and attachment. A love without demands and expectations. This is the purest form of love where you give of yourself to others rather than trying to fulfill your own needs. Unconditional love never uses or abuses. It is true compassion in expression.

RESPONSIBILITY: You have total responsibility for who you are, your own actions, and well-being. Nobody but you can change the situation you have put yourself in. What you do to others, good or bad, will inevitably come back to yourself. Respect this Law of Cause and Effect and take full responsibility for your own actions. In this way you can create a more harmonious life for yourself by giving in kindness to others.

SURRENDER: Do what you can to find the solutions to your problems. Take responsibility for them, but then let them go. Surrender and trust in the universal flow of wisdom and love. Trust that you are a perfect being right here and now. Everything that comes to you is for your highest good, and for your optimal growth on all levels. Expect the very best, but do not establish any limitations by deciding what it is you want. The Universe will always provide your needs. Trust that everything happens in your best interest, even if it is not what you had planned or wished for. The Universe has no limitations. When opening your heart in surrender, it will give you more than you would ever dream of. Do not limit the Universe! Surrender—and live in trust.

GRATITUDE: Look around you. Really look! See and experience all that is yours. Be grateful for who you are. Be grateful for everything you have. Give thanks for all the experiences and lessons you have been given. Deep inside your being feel the warmth of gratitude to the greatness of life. For the fact that you exist, and that you are here to express— in the here and now.

REIKI AND YOUR POWER WITHIN

The Reiki initiations increase the awareness, and thereby prepare us for further expansion and growth. The Reiki energy radiating from the hands is merely a side-effect of the initiation process, which sets up the means for further unfoldment and growth. Reiki expands the ability to think, understand and accept. It becomes easier to find our own path and philosophy of life. Reiki helps in developing inner strength that brings us forward, and that gives us power to go on when the road gets tough. Without inner strength we risk being ruled by other people's ideas rather than following our own inner voice. If we are not trusting our own inner knowledge, which often is the case in the beginning, it is easy to believe that others know more or have come further in their development than ourselves. We forget, or have not yet realized, that the truth is hidden in our own hearts. Instead we listen to other people's opinions, and perhaps uncritically jump from one idea to the next, believing we can find the answer to our inner yearning through external factors.

Reiki is one technique that puts us in touch with our own worth and the hidden wisdom within. Reiki expands intuition, creativity and intellect, and strengthens the link between the ego and the higher self. Reiki aids in the process of reclaiming our own life by listening within, realizing that truth dwells inside of ourselves and not with others. The world consists of as many truths as there are people on earth. Each one of us hold our own world view. What is right for others does not have to be right for you. Do not limit yourself with the belief that somebody else is higher, more advanced or knows more about spiritual and esoteric matters than you do. When you are in contact with your higher self *you* have all the answers at hand!

Today there are many different movements, teachings and ideas around. It is impossible to follow everything new that comes your way. Use discrimination, and be careful not to become a seminar junkie because of your own insecurity. The supply is tremendous and there are seminars on just about everything. To indiscriminately attend one seminar after the other only leads to an endless and unfulfilled search. Understand that truth and wholeness cannot be found outside of yourself. It is by going within, listening to the inner voice, that true peace and harmony will be found. Nobody can fill our inner void for us from the outside, regardless of how many courses we attend, how many organizations we belong to, or how much we read about and listen to other people's ideas about life and universal truth.

Before you take on somebody else's ideas, ask yourself if they feel right for you. If you get an uneasy feeling, or sense that something may be wrong, listen to that inner voice! All the truth and wisdom lays within you. All you need to do is develop your ability to listen. You do not need to go to psychics or mediums. You do not need to accept what other people say, just because they "have come so far". Why give away the right to your own life to somebody else? There is no reason to let somebody else decide your future or how you should feel. Just because it superficially seems as though someone else has a greater knowledge than you, it does not necessarily have to be so. Nobody knows you, or your situation, better than you do. If you follow your inner voice you will be right, no matter what others might say or think about the subject. By listening within you develop discrimination. You learn that whatever you feel in your heart is right for you. Anything else can be ignored. It does not have to be part of your world unless you choose it to be. Follow the road you have started to travel. The way may become much longer if you turn at every crossroads, and there is a risk that you forget your purpose, or delay your journey forward in life.

At the same time as it is important to know your own worth and listen to your internal knowledge, it is also important that you stay open to your surroundings not rejecting what you meet without investigation. To find your own way in life you must first become aware of what you have around you. Give what you see, hear or meet a chance, but listen carefully to your inner voice before adopting the new. Be aware there may be things that are questionable in the jungle of new and old movements and ideas trying to catch an eager seeker's attention. If you are told about demands, stipulations and rules, or that you must act this way or that—beware! On the way through life *you* are both the actor and the director. You do not have to follow the opinions and rules made by somebody else. The rules and laws of society are naturally a different matter. Of course we follow the written Law to prevent total chaos and anarchy to break out, but be careful if somebody tries to manipulate you onto a way that you feel in your heart is not the right one for you.

Somebody might tell you that in order to develop you must first give up all your belongings. If so, listen to the alarm bells going off in your inner. There is no Universal Law that stipulates that we must suffer, be poor, hungry, grovel in the dust and be without self-respect, to be able to grow spiritually. In fact, the reverse is true! If you respect and love yourself, you will respect and love others, and you can give unconditionally. By giving of yourself in a loving way, you emit positive energy into the Universe, and positive energy will thereby be attracted to you. (That is a Universal Law.) Life will be easier to live and you will have more love and energy leftover to others. You will therefore experience more abundance and love in your own life. This is true unfoldment. The human being is not meant to stagnate in rules, demands, manipulation and have-to's, stipulated and established by somebody claiming to be a spiritual being, guru or founder of some particular movement or association.

Be open but not naive to life. We can learn immensely from each other. Every person possesses a fantastic storage of knowledge and wisdom. Listening and learning from others is part of our growth process. That does not mean you let low self-worth fool you to believe you know less. It does not mean that everything you hear from others must be right and better than what you have. Listen to other people's ideas with interest, but maintain your own world view until the new you are told really proves to give more joy and success than what you already have. Respect other people's opinions and feelings about themselves and their situation. Remember that what feels right for them is their absolute truth. Who are you to question that? Allow others to have their truths. Respect their ideas and opinions so that you will have the freedom to keep your own identity. Defend your right of integrity only if somebody tries to give you his truth in an interfering or unethical way. Be assured that all you do is absolutely right for you, regardless of the opinions others might have about your choices and way of living. Your way is yours, and you can never travel the way of another. Sometimes we might travel together, helping and supporting each other at difficult stretches of the road. We can give compassion and understanding to somebody who struggles uphill by our side. By understanding and helping this fellow being, we may begin to fill our own inner, and find love and truth in life.

SIX

REIKI TREATMENTS

*R*eiki is a technique that helps in making peoples' lives easier, but like all other tools it doesn't work if we choose not to use the aid offered. To achieve optimal health on all levels it is necessary to apply Reiki regularly. Reiki has the same function as food or sleep. We constantly need to fill up the stores, since we are in continual use of the energy supplied. You cannot give Reiki during one period of your life and then assume you would not need any more thinking you have filled up the store. Just like you need to eat and sleep daily in order to cope, you will feel better and have more energy if you make Reiki a part of your daily life.

TREATMENT OF YOURSELF

By far the most important aspect of Reiki is treating yourself. Reiki allows you to take control of your own state of health and well-being on all levels. By giving yourself Reiki daily you establish the format of your own preventive health care. You maximize your health-potential and quicken your emotional, intellectual and spiritual development. You also actively treat all physical manifestations of lacking health, symptoms and diseases that have accumulated until today.

To maximize the benefits of Reiki, you set aside one uninterrupted hour each day. This hour will be spent in solitude, treating yourself. Some people believe they do not have any spare time for themselves. They live in the belief they are not worthy of one single hour out of the day's twenty-four. If we do not make use of the help and tools we have around us it is often due to lack of self worth. We do not appreciate ourselves and our own excellence. Instead of using the unique opportunity Reiki provides, we unconsciously try to sabotage our own healing, both physically and emotionally. Subconsciously we feel that we are not worthy of health and well-being. In the same way as our lower self can sabotage every attempt to improvement in our career and social life, we can also sabotage our own healing and further development.

After having Reiki activated in your body systems the most important step is treating yourself. If you give yourself the gift of Reiki every day you will experience dramatic changes, both within yourself and in those around you. You will feel better for each day, as will the people around you, and as a consequence your life will start to change. This course of events will be initiated by the new, more harmonious energies you radiate. The hour you spend looking after and caring for yourself will reward you with better self-confidence, inner strength, more energy and a stronger physical body. Giving yourself Reiki is a marvelous way of giving love and care to yourself, and to develop a sound relationship to your body and person.

In the long term you actually do not lose any time in treating yourself. The truth is that you gain time by setting aside this daily hour for yourself and your own well-being. One hour of Reiki treatment equals three to four hours of deep sleep regarding increased oxygen supply to the blood stream, cell repair, tissue renewal, and general rejuvenation of the body. Your sleep becomes deeper and more restful, and thus you do not need to sleep as many hours as you used to. Personally I have decreased my sleep requirement from nine hours to approximately six or seven hours per night since taking up Reiki. I wake up fully rested; still in bed I give myself an hour of Reiki, and this leaves me full of energy to meet the new day. Furthermore, I have also gained a couple of extra hours of awake time.

Of course Reiki is no substitute for sleep, but it can be used as a very good supplement for increased vitality and health. Sleep is obviously a too important part of the human nature to be replaced by Reiki or anything else. To be able to stay sound we need regular sleep and uninterrupted periods of dreams. Dream scientists have shown that people deprived of their dream time, a couple of nights in a row, start to hallucinate and show serious psychological disturbances. Dreams help us to catalogue events and sort out the experiences we have had during the day. Sleep is important to our mental health but most people sleep more than necessary due to a restless and scattered sleep pattern. Reiki helps us utilize our day better by giving us a deeper, more restful but shorter sleep.

Many people suffer from sleep deficiency due to many years of sleep deprivation. They have an accumulated need for catching up on sleep. If this is the case it might take a few weeks of regular treatments or longer before experiencing any benefits of Reiki. During this time the treatments might even cause more tiredness and need of sleep. This is the body's natural way of catching up and regaining strength and vitality.

Immediately when starting to use Reiki the body will begin to heal itself from many different imbalances, both known and unknown, that might have been harbored for years. This initiated healing process is another reason for the possible need of even more sleep in the early stages of experiencing Reiki. The body simply heals more effectively when asleep. Reiki treats illnesses and disturbances in the body long before we are aware of any physical problems. This is also true for serious illnesses. Even if a person is totally unaware of a serious condition, he or she may experience an increased need for sleep during a number of weeks, months or even years after starting regular treatments of Reiki. To most people three weeks of daily Reiki treatments seem to be sufficient to start experiencing a lower requirement for sleep, as well as other positive changes in body and mind.

After the Reiki attunements, the body sometimes counter-reacts with a so-called healing crisis. Reiki creates harmony in an unbalanced body system, and initiates or accelerates a healing process where so needed. The body's first attempt to achieve health may in some cases be experienced as momentarily increased pain in already damaged areas or areas with chronic pain. This pain normally lasts for only a short period, and it is a good sign that the injury or problem is actively healing. However, in a few cases the pain has been known to last for as long as up to a year. It is mostly chronic pain that might lead to this condition. When released the pain is usually gone for good.

In the initial stages of Reiki some discomfort may be experienced due to the cleansing process that is triggered. The physical detoxification normally lasts for a day or two, and is typically experienced as light to severe headaches, nausea and/or diarrhea. Psychologically the detoxification is expressed in the form of mood swings, where different emotions such as crying, anger fits and laughter may appear. These reactions are not to be interpreted as negative side-effects, but as the body's positive, natural and healthy detoxification process. The body reacts in a similar way as in the beginning of a fast, i.e., with a substantial cleaning out of toxic matter that has gathered in the body over the years, both physically and psychologically. This is a very positive reaction, that eventually leads to increased well-being when some of the physical and emotional baggage has been discarded. The emotional cleansing process tends to go on a bit longer than the physical.

You may experience the first three weeks after the Reiki activation as an adjustment period. It is a time of purge and detoxification, and getting to know the new energy in the body. During these weeks you may at times, but not necessarily, experience some physical discomfort and upset or confused emotions. It is important that you give yourself some extra time and nurturing during these weeks. Take care of yourself and don't put yourself under too much stress. Try to let things pass by without letting it affect you, and give yourself plenty of time for your daily Reiki treatment.

During these first weeks it is very important that you make sure to give yourself Reiki every day. You are establishing a new habit, where Reiki takes a place in your life, and you adjust to fit it into your everyday lifestyle. Furthermore, regular Reiki treatments give you a better chance to really experience changes and improvements in yourself and your body.

HEAD	FRONT	BACK
position 1	position 5	position 9
position 2	position 6	position 10
position 3	position 7	position 11
position 4	position 8	position 12

During my seminars I strongly recommend all the students to really make sure they give themselves one full hour of Reiki every day for the first three weeks. I tell them to do their Reiki even if they have to sacrifice something else for it. I want them to do Reiki also when they do not feel like it and have to force themselves to get started. The subconscious mind works diligently to maintain control, and it dreads all news that promise change. It feels immediately threatened by all techniques and methods that lead to increased awareness and further growth, and it defends itself by constantly whispering in our ear that we don't have to do it today. It doesn't matter if it is about Reiki, new eating habits, new exercise program, or something else. The internal little saboteur will whisper compellingly that we can always start tomorrow. The problem, of course, is that tomorrow never comes. Be aware of this self sabotaging trait and try to overcome it by practicing discipline. Work on creating a new habit involving daily Reiki treatments.

However, Reiki should of course not be perceived as another "have-to". We are not supposed to sigh over the need of having to do Reiki, or that we must squeeze another hour into our already hectic schedule. To give Reiki is to give the gift of peace and harmony, nurturing, care and love to yourself. After a few weeks of regular treatments a positive need of taking care of yourself, to relax and to release accumulated stress, is often created. After passing the threshold of internal resistance you will be looking forward to your daily hour. Therefore, make sure that you use Reiki every day for the first three weeks, irrespective of how you feel about it. After giving Reiki a fair chance you can make up your mind about whether you want to continue or not. Usually you would already feel the benefits of Reiki by now; you sleep better, need less sleep, are more alert, more rested and if you previously had any kind of pain it probably has lessened. You have most likely managed to fit Reiki in at a time that fits your daily routine, and are now able continue with your hour without much trouble. The secret to getting started is to persist in working with your treatments during the initial period.

The intention is to continue with Reiki also after the first three weeks, but never make Reiki a compulsory drag. We have enough have-to's in our lives and we don't need to add more. The world is not going to fall apart if you don't give yourself a treatment. Have a break that day without any guilt. Fanaticism is never healthy. Common sense must be used in all we do. To skip a Reiki treatment now and then is not going to hurt. It is when you realize that several days or weeks have passed without Reiki that it is time to be aware. Your internal saboteur has taken control again. Remember then, that you have control over your own life. You can at any moment choose to once more take up Reiki to enhance your health and well-being. You have responsibility for your own state of health, and it is only your own insecurity and self-contempt that allows you to stray from the techniques and tools that can help you live a better and healthier life.

It could be an interesting experience to keep a journal during the first weeks with Reiki. It helps you keep track of what is happening to your health and to become aware of any changes and improvements in your life. Start with writing down a present health report and how you see yourself and your situation right now. Write about your social life, work, family, any illnesses and problems, etc., including everything around you and your emotional state. Write about the things you are not happy with, but also the changes you would like to see come in to you life. Writing about the things we want to change, exclude or add to our lives, helps convert abstract dreams to realistic goals. To set objectives is an important part of successful peoples' lives. There is no secret to these peoples' success. Achievements come from focused work and intent, that steadily leads to a pre-set destination. People who have set and determined goals, and who are not set back by adversity, will achieve the most in life. They know how to achieve what they set out to do and how to fulfill their dreams and goals. The difference between success and failure lay in the strength of continuously keeping the vision of the goal clear and distinct in your mind, and to actively work towards its realization. But remember that success has less to do with money and material wealth than with joy, love, sense of belonging and health. Goal-setting is of course not specific to Reiki, but utilizing the promise of a new beginning that Reiki offers, right in the middle of the life that you already lead, can be as good a start as any. Not everyone is given the chance to take part in such an opportunity, so grab it and start now to actively realize your dreams by writing them down, thus turning them into substantial goals.

Another interesting aspect of writing about your life as it is right now, is that you can later compare and notice the changes that have occurred. If you don't do this, it might be easy to forget or ignore the changes you have accomplished. Six months or a year down the track you might have forgotten how difficult your situation was, what pain you were in, or how often you were ill before you started using Reiki. If you have written everything down, you can remind yourself, and really become aware of the achievements. It is hard to look at yourself objectively, hence you will be the last one to notice your own improvements. On a subtle level others will be aware of your more balanced behavior long before yourself, and they will automatically treat you in a new and more harmonious manner. You can use these people's different way of treating you as a measurement of your own development. The more friends and acquaintances you meet that seem to have gone through a positive change, the more you can be certain of your own growth.

Your change cannot be perceived from one day to another. You will need to give both yourself and Reiki time. It takes continuance for changes to occur because our physical existence is of a very high density and it is therefore slow to move. This time-delay provides the means for developing patience and persistence, but it also enhances our ability to surrender and allow the universal energy to flow without our limited, personal involvement. Despite the high density and inertia of our physical universe I am constantly surprised by how quickly some people manage to create a new life and a new reality for themselves after participating in a Reiki seminar.

During the First Degree Seminar you will be taught how to give yourself Reiki treatments. You work according to a simple schedule, where you learn how to place your hands in twelve different positions on your body (see page 81). You stay for approximately five minutes in each position and the entire treatment takes more or less an hour. Do not become too fixated by the clock, since this will interfere with your relaxation. You do not need to constantly check how much time you have left. Intuitively you will soon feel approximately when the five minutes are up and it is time to move on to the next position. Initially you can for example go through the four positions of the head and then look at the clock to get an idea of how you are doing with time. You can then do four more positions before checking the time again. That way you will soon get a feeling for how long to stay in each position. You may also record a cassette tape with relaxing music with five minutes intervals. Your voice or a bell can let you know when it is time to move your hands. Both CD's and audio-tapes, with five minute pieces of relaxing music and nature sounds, can be ordered. See details at the back of the book. For most people however, the timing is not a problem.

It doesn't matter if you happen to spend seven minutes in one place and three in another. What matters is that you actually give yourself Reiki. Learn to listen to and trust your own hands. The hand positions you learn in the seminar are only recommendations. They are developed to cover the most vital organs and Chakras of the body, but if you feel that you want to place your hands on another area, or if you want to stay for a longer or shorter period in one place, you should follow your intuition and do so. Nobody knows your body as well as you. Your hands know where Reiki is needed and are automatically drawn there. Don't fight the natural flow, just be flexible within your treatment.

Make sure that you are not going to be interrupted when you give yourself a treatment. Do not lie in front of the TV, for example. It is disturbing, and if a violent or aggressive program is on you may become negatively affected to a greater extent than if you were awake. We do not need more and deeper negative programming than what we are already involuntarily exposed to every day.

You can give yourself Reiki at any time of the day, and anywhere you want to be, but the best place would probably be in bed. Many people do their Reiki just before they go to sleep at night or before they get up in the morning. These times are good as the demands of the day are over or have not yet started. To give yourself the treatment at any of these times will make it easier for you to comfortably fit Reiki into your life. If you give yourself Reiki at a time when other people think you are sleeping, the risk of being disturbed during the treatment is lessened as well.

Reiki is a very simple technique to use. All you have to do is be sufficiently awake to place your hands in the first body position and you are on your way. You will then drift in and out of a very relaxed stage moving your hands at appropriate times. If possible, put your hands on your naked skin. If you have problems accepting yourself and your body it could be a very powerful experience to, as a change, touch yourself lovingly rather than the usual abuse of indifference, harsh words or disgust. Make sure you are comfortable during the treatment. Support your arms with pillows where necessary in order for you to relax. You might fall asleep at times during your treatment and that is okay too. Just complete the treatment on awakening. If you are late and have to get up immediately you may finish the treatment at another time. The most common reason for falling asleep during the treatment is the body's need of more Reiki in that position. The hands will then be left in that same position until you wake up or involuntarily move, and the body gets Reiki exactly where needed even as you sleep. Try to become aware of where your hands are positioned when falling asleep. It will usually be in the same position each time, indicating a greater need for Reiki in that place of your body. Give yourself extra Reiki in that area during the day. As you achieve greater harmony and balance in the body energies, the need for extra Reiki in particular places will decrease.

Reiki is attracted to the areas where it is needed the most and where the greatest imbalances are located, irrespective of where your hands are placed on the body. In theory this would mean the hands could be held in one position during the entire treatment and the energy would still flow to the areas of imbalance and disease. Although this is correct it does not quite work like that in reality since most people have blockages and disturbances in the flow of energy in various places of their bodies. If we have a serious problem that needs lot's of Reiki and we place the hands far away from that particular area, some of the energy will be attracted to blockages and imbalances along the way, as they too need to be cleared. Treating locally, i.e. right on the area of injury or disease, is therefore important in helping the healing process and to achieve the best and quickest results. This is the reason why we place our hands in twelve different positions on the body when treating ourselves or somebody else with Reiki.

The energy flow of Reiki will be stronger if you stay aware of what you are doing, i.e. that your focus is on the treatment and your hands, but Reiki does not require any extreme concentration to work. Just idly observing what is going on in your body during the treatment is sufficient for a full flow. Do not become overly fixed on what you are doing since that would disturb your relaxation. Allow your thoughts to drift without trying to force them back. It is normal that your mind is activated and your thoughts wander during the treatment. This is a consequence of the healing and cleansing process that Reiki initiates. Relax completely but also keep a subtle awareness of your Reiki. Your intent of giving Reiki is the important action.

Reiki is not a meditation technique, and therefore does not need any particular concentration or other internal activity in order to work. The only thing required is that you consciously place your hands on the body. Then you just have to allow the energy to flow as it pleases. You will, however, automatically fall into a very deep relaxation similar to what is achieved in meditation. After about ten minutes into the treatment your brain frequency has slowed down to Alpha level, i.e. the same relaxed state as an experienced meditator achieves. You will reach the Alpha level relaxation without any active cooperation on your part. After approximately another thirty minutes into the treatment you reach an even deeper state of relaxation called the Theta level. This is the deepest relaxed state possible to achieve and still maintain consciousness. The next state of brain frequency is called the Delta level and is equal to being unconscious or in a very deep sleep. The brain vibrates in Beta frequency when awake and alert. Spending some time in the Theta level is very good for our health. The Theta level offers a very deep relaxation, where lot's of natural and effective healing occurs. In our stressed-out society it is important to find time for deep rest and peace of mind on a daily basis, in order not to be torn apart by all the demands and pressures we are facing. Reiki offers a simple technique for reaching deep relaxation without requiring any extensive practice or education.

It is important trying to keep the entire treatment in one section because we relax more deeply as the hour goes on. Of course our body system receives as much Reiki if we choose to do two half hour sessions during the day, or three twenty minute sessions, but we lose the deep relaxation and the effective natural healing the complete hour provides. Therefore, do not split your Reiki hour unless it is absolutely necessary and you have very special reasons. If you make it a habit to give yourself the whole hour uninterrupted, you will experience deeper rest and a clearer mind as time goes on. Reiki offers an effective stress release, and since many of today's illnesses and problems are stress related, Reiki is of great value for both physical and mental well-being. By giving yourself regular treatments you will not be affected to the same extent by the daily stress factors. You will also find it easier to take control of your situation and to take responsibility for the decisions you make.

Sometimes memories surface during or after a Reiki treatment, because the mind is activated during the deep relaxation. The memories stirred may reveal difficult experiences, that have been suppressed for a long time, due to the pain they caused. Also memories of pleasant events that make you happy and content might be recalled. Memories come forward because they need to be dealt with. The issue might be painful, but remembering may be necessary in order to let go of what has been and to be able to move on. Previous experiences that have not been appropriately dealt with can have such a strong hold over us that we stagnate and stop our growth process. They can make us feel very bad in our present situation. Reiki never brings forth more than we can handle at this moment, and there is never any risk that we would not be able to handle whatever surfaces. Be prepared to release the energy in these memories by crying, laughing, screaming and raving, or with any other emotional expression.

Remembering may be an important part of the healing process, but at other times it is not necessary to actively recall a particular event. Many incidents are assimilated internally, and this can be physically noticed in the stomach area. Release of memories and suppressed emotions are experienced as more or less loud rumblings from the belly area. Other ways of releasing memories, experiences, and suppressed feelings stored in the physical body are little spasms in small muscle groups, primarily in the arms, legs and face, similar to what we experience just before falling asleep. The muscle tightens, and is then released with a sudden jerk as the emotional energy is discharged.

Each person reacts to Reiki in their own way. Everyone therefore has to experiment with the treatments to find the best suitable time for themselves. Some get a real boost of energy immediately after the treatment. For these people the best time for treating themselves would be early in the morning before getting out of bed. Initially it might be necessary to set the alarm one hour earlier than usual to get started, but the body will soon adjust and awake at the right time. Other people feel so relaxed and cozy after the treatment that they will happily roll over and fall asleep. For them going through the program before falling asleep at night would be most appropriate. You have to find out what feels best for you. Maybe you will even change after a while and switch from evening to morning or vice versa. Timing is just a practical detail and is obviously of no importance to the effect of the treatment.

You can use every opportunity to give yourself extra Reiki during the day by making it a habit of always letting your hands rest in a comfortable position on the body whenever you have any spare time. You may use these moments for treating particular parts of the body and areas with problems or pain. You can use one or both of your hands when giving extra Reiki. In this way you will always be using your time efficiently. You may for instance give yourself Reiki when you are in a meeting, in the car, in a bus, or in front of the TV. If you give Reiki with one hand, you will obviously receive only half as much energy as if you were using both of your hands. The extra Reiki helps in strengthening and speeding up the final result, but since your mind is distracted by other activities you will not experience the same deep relaxation as you do during a full treatment laying down. The Reiki you give when you are busy doing something else will not be as strong as when you consciously are giving yourself a treatment.

You can give yourself several treatments a day if you are very ill or in discomfort. Your body will draw exactly as much energy as it needs, which makes Reiki impossible to overdose. If you are in bed, whether at home or in the hospital, you can give yourself several hours of Reiki each day to help speed up your recovery. You might start with going through the twelve positions. After completing the treatment you may just let your hands rest in a comfortable position or the area of pain, allowing the energy to flow freely.

The systematic treatment of the entire body is important to your optimal well-being. However, injuries less that twenty-four hours old should always be treated locally. Emergencies and accidents are treated immediately by placing the hands directly on the injury, or an inch above if there is an open would or the area is very sore to touch. If this is the case you may also place your hands right beside the injury.

Small problems like minor burns, cuts and abrasions can easily be fixed with Reiki, and normally no other treatment is necessary. More serious injuries, however, should always be treated by a physician. While waiting for the doctor or ambulance you can alleviate pain, stop the flow of blood, prevent shock and dramatically speed up the healing process by giving Reiki. You will of course continue to give Reiki after the visit to the doctor or in the hospital. Remember that the energy penetrates almost anything, for example plasters and thin layers of metal.

Trust your hands and make a habit of always placing them on any injuries you might attract to yourself. It is never wrong or dangerous to use Reiki! As long as you use common sense, not thinking you can fix serious injuries without seeing a physician, you will have great help from the pain-relief and enhanced healing Reiki offers. There will be many times when you can save yourself a trip to the physician if the accident is minor, but do not act stupidly. If you are in the least uncertain, you should immediately call your doctor or go to the hospital to have your injury examined and treated!

Reiki speeds up the healing dramatically, and in many cases the injury might be almost completely healed by the time you reach the hospital, but it is still better to go one time too many just to be on the safe side.

Some people think Reiki is too good to be true, but that is usually an illusionary understanding. The technique is very simple and no special knowledge or training is required. Even small children can learn how to use the simple principles, but this does not mean Reiki is easy. A great deal of self-discipline is required in order to make full use of the advantages of Reiki. The weak link, when neglecting to care for oneself, is often the convenience-orientation of the human mind. The technological society of today has spoiled us, and we expect results without making any effort of our own. Reiki does not work that way. We must actively use the technique Reiki offers in order for it to improve our lives. Unfortunately many people choose to take medicines or go through major surgery, rather than making long term changes to their lifestyle. Thousands of people die every year because they refused to follow simple recommendations from their physician, such as giving up smoking, improving their eating habits, and/or starting to exercise. Unfortunately, Reiki falls into the same category. It is easier to let somebody else fix our problems with surgery or pills, than to give ourselves one hour of Reiki treatment a day.

To improve our lives and health from the core we need to take responsibility for how we feel, and to make conscious changes. This cannot happen if we placidly wait for somebody else to fix our lives for us. We must actively make the decision of using Reiki, to improve our lives and strengthen our health potential. Nothing is for free. We must treat ourselves to one hour of Reiki every day to achieve its optimal effect. Particularly in the beginning, time and effort are needed in order to experience the advantages, but the results achieved are well worth the effort. Not until you take responsibility for your life will you actively start your own growth process.

TREATMENTS OF OTHERS

In this section I will call the person receiving Reiki the client, and the person giving the treatment the practitioner.

When treating others it is important to maintain your detachment, and not to expect particular results. If you are fixed on a particular result, i.e. a specific recovery, through expectations or hope or because of your ego, you risk not only to be disappointed since Reiki is drawn to where it is needed the most and not to where you want it, you also open yourself to negative energies. If you try to achieve results according to your own will, by forcing yourself on the natural flow, you interfere with a greater plan and in some way you are trying to bargain with God. It might at times be very tempting to wish a sick person well, but we have absolutely no right to interfere in any other way than by the service and practical help we can give. The rest needs to be surrendered to a greater power than ours.

It is a spiritual infringement to pray, send light, or try to affect the recovery of a sick person in other metaphysical ways without that persons clear consent. Illnesses are part of the learning process and something everyone must go through on their own in order to unfold and move on. This is true also when the person has to leave the physical body behind in order to continue the journey in another dimension. If we stop, or interfere, with that process we meddle with another person's life in an unethical way. By not allowing the person to go through, and learn from his illnesses and problems, we risk taking them on in his place.

If you maintain your detachment of the final result, also when it is not what you wished for or planned, there is no risk in giving Reiki to other's. If you still want to protect yourself further, picture yourself in a bubble of white or blue light before starting the treatment.

Visualize how the swirling light surrounds your body. Become aware of the strength and protection it provides. Feel yourself absolutely safe inside of your own impenetrable ball of light. Ask for the will of God to be done, not your own, by quietly stating: "Thy will be done". Remove your ego from the scene.

Remember, detachment is not the same as being indifferent and cold. It is much easier to give unconditional love and compassion to another fellow being when one is not tied down by strings of opinions and expectations. Also understand that feeling sorry for another person will only place this person below yourself. From your place of pity you look down at this unfortunate person and his misery. You are automatically placing yourself in a superior position by doing this. True healing cannot take place in such an imbalanced environment.

Do everything in your power to help a fellow human being, particularly when ill. Take care of practical details and give service. Give as much Reiki as you can, but do not try to direct the energy in any particular way because that is not possible. If you let your ego get in the way, you only risk to open yourself to somebody else's burdens. Stay in your power, be compassionate, do not fall for the temptation of trying to direct the end result of Reiki, and you will experience many good moments together with your clients.

Always give a full hour of Reiki unless you are dealing with emergencies. Treat locally, i.e., directly on the injury, up to twenty-four hours after an accident. The sooner you can treat an emergency, the quicker and better the healing. Do not wait! Put your hands on the injury immediately and keep them there for thirty to forty minutes or more, depending on the type and size of the impairment. Smaller injuries require less time, while more serious ones can be treated for several hours, if need be. Use your common sense and intuition, and you will "know" when enough Reiki has been given.

It is quite common that smaller problems like headaches and different aches and pains disappear with only a short boost of Reiki, but do not make a habit out of giving "quickie" treatments of five to ten minutes. It is nice that Reiki often gives swift relief, but in the event of a more serious problem the "quickie" might not work and the client and others involved may get the wrong impression of Reiki. It is often due to these "quickies" that Reiki is misunderstood. This is a pity as Reiki is proven to effectively speed up the body's natural healing process. Sometimes the symptoms disappear quickly, but to achieve a deep and lasting healing more Reiki than just a few minutes must be allowed. Some people, cynically or devotedly, try to give Reiki magical properties, but Reiki does not fall into the category of extra-terrestrial powers, spells or magic. Reiki is an energy with powerful healing abilities, and as such requires time and effort to work optimally.

Make sure people understand the difference between a short sample of Reiki and a full body treatment. If you are only going to give a few minutes of Reiki, then explain that this is not a complete treatment, but there is still a good possibility Reiki will offer temporary relief. A simple rule is: A lot of Reiki is better that a little Reiki. A little Reiki is better than no Reiki.

Best, of course, is to give the client a complete treatment, covering the entire body (see page 95). This will take sixty to seventy minutes. You place your hands in twelve different positions and stay for approximately five minutes in each spot. Give three treatments shortly after one another, each or every second day is good. You will thereby strengthen the healing curve and the client will recover more rapidly. The first three treatments should preferably be given within a week. This is to kick start the process, and to give Reiki optimal effect in strengthening and healing the body. Decide on three appointment dates at once, before meeting for the first treatment. If the client does not want to receive more than one treatment, despite your information that it normally is necessary to receive several treatments for maximum results, this is the client's own choice. The client thereby accepts responsibility for the end result. Understand this important ethic as it will help eliminate the risk of you placing specific expectations on the outcome. It will also prevent you from taking the results you and your client achieve together, or the times when Reiki has seemingly no visible effect, personally.

HEAD	FRONT	BACK
position 1	position 5	position 9

| position 2 | position 6 | position 10 |

| position 3 | position 7 | position 11 |

| position 4 | position 8 | position 12 |

Remember that you are not Reiki. All you contribute during a treatment is your hands that you lend for a little more that an hour at the time. Reiki flows through your hands, but you are not the energy. Reiki is *automatically* drawn to areas of imbalance, and your task is solely to be with the client, hold you hands still on his body and allow the energy transference to take place.

After the first three sessions you continue to give regular treatments once or twice a week until the problem or illness is gone. The length of time between treatments is of course related to the nature of the illness and to practicality. A seriously ill person can receive several treatments a day, while a person having treatments for personal development, stress release, preventive care or the like, can get by on one treatment a week or less depending on how quickly one wants to see results. It is of course always most effective to activate Reiki in your own body at a First Degree Reiki seminar. You will thereby receive constant and continuous access to the energy at all times. Furthermore, working with Reiki yourself is a good way to reclaim responsibility for your own health and lessen your dependency on other people. However, the attunement process can only be performed by a trained Reiki Master.

Give the Reiki treatments in a quiet place, preferably in a room where you can close the door and where you will not be interrupted. If you are treating from home, let the rest of the family know that they cannot disturb you when you are with a client. Unplug the telephone or switch over to the answering machine before starting.

If you do not own a massage table, the client can simply lie on an ordinary kitchen table covered by a mattress or a folded duvet. Avoid converting a bed into a treatment table. If you sit on the edge of the bed, you have to twist your back in an awkward position to be able to reach, and you might be terribly uncomfortable. You might place your client on a mattress on the floor, but then you need to sit with your arms in the same static position for five minutes in each position for a whole hour or more. It can be very difficult to do this comfortably when sitting on the floor. For your own comfort a table of some sort is recommended.

It is important that you sit or stand comfortably when giving Reiki treatments or you may develop pains in your own body, particularly in back, shoulders and neck. Any tension you might experience is also transferred to your client, who senses your discomfort and restlessness, and is therefore unable to relax properly.

Encourage the client to loosen any tight clothing before starting the treatment. Open up at the neck, loosen the belt, the bra, etc. The client can remain fully clothed since Reiki passes through fabric, leather, plaster and other materials. Make the client comfortable by putting a pillow under the knees when on his back. Move the pillow under the ankles when turning over to the belly.

If the client suffers from back pain, you may try placing a pillow under the hips when face down to ease the strain. Let women late in pregnancy lay on their sides, since they might pass out in a supine position. Support with pillows where needed for relaxation and comfort. It is common that the body's temperature drops slightly during the treatment and the client might start to feel cold. Keep a blanket nearby so you do not have to leave your client during the treatment.

Explain in simple ways what is going to occur during the treatment before you start: Your are using your hands to supply a harmonious energy that will enable the body to heal itself, and which will restore the body's depleted energy resources. Tell your client that you will stay by his side once you have initiated the treatment. Show the different hand positions you will use. Start by placing your hands over the face and ask the client if that feels okay. Ask the client to close his eyes and relax. The client will soon sink into a deep meditative state where he is more open and sensitive than normally.

Internal reactions, memories and emotions within the client create a unique experience, and the only contact with the external world is your warm hands that pleasantly rest on the body. Therefore, *do not* leave your client once you have started the treatment! The person you are treating is feeling trust and comfort in your hands. Always leave one hand on the client to inspire safety, also when turning the client over or moving your hands to a new position.

Many of the previous traumas and unfinished business stored within will be resolved on a deeper level, beyond the conscious mind. Do not disturb this process by talking! If the client needs to express any memories that might surface, then listen without interfering. Be aware that some people may be afraid of confronting their own inner depth. The client reaches a deeper contact with himself and the Reiki treatment might seem threatening at first. Instead of relaxing, eyes closed, the client might follow all your movements with wide open eyes, or talk himself through the treatment. Do not encourage a chit-chat conversation by involving yourself in a discussion. Ask the client once more to close his eyes, relax and try to go with the treatment. After a few treatments even those who initially are very worried will be able to relax. It is not difficult to separate the chit-chat from a deep inner experience that the client needs to share. In the event of the latter you will of course allow the client to talk without interrupting. Whether the client has his eyes closed or open, talks or is quiet, he will receive the same amount of Reiki. What is lost through talking is the deep relaxation, stress relief and inner understanding that are usually experienced during a totally relaxed Reiki treatment. Playing meditative music may be good in helping the client relax.

During the treatment you will either follow the schedule with the twelve different positions or your own intuition. Trust the feelings in your hands. Rest the weight of your arms and hands lightly on the client, that feels nice and nurturing and is not experienced as heavy. Be careful when treating face and neck, which are more sensitive to touch than the rest of the body. Finish off by holding the feet for a couple of minutes to stabilize and ground the client. You might lightly massage the feet in order to gently alert the client.

You do not need to wave your hands over the client, pull energies, or do other movements over the body when finished. Magnetic healing, polarity healing and some other forms of laying on of hands require the right techniques to correctly finish off a treatment. In completing these kind of treatments the subtle energies around the body might need to be balanced by the practitioner's pulling, moving and/or removing. These types of healing work are using the body's own physical or magnetic energies, therefore it is necessary to make certain maneuvers afterwards to "close up", and to balance and conserve the energy. It is known that well-intentioned people have confused Reiki with other types of body therapies, and some of these finishing-off techniques have unnecessarily been added to Reiki. These techniques have subsequently been taught to others as an essential part of the Reiki treatment. It is important to understand that this is a completely unnecessary activity. The energy flow of Reiki starts as soon as the hands are placed on the body, and stops as soon as they are removed. We neither open nor close anything in the body's energy fields when giving Reiki, and there is therefore no need to be waving about in the subtle energies and/or rubbing the body in different ways as a completion of the treatment. All you need to do when finishing off a treatment is to remove your hands, tell your client the treatment is over, and allow appropriate time to wake up from the deep relaxation.

Make sure you have some spare time after the treatment in case the client has a need to talk about experiences and memories that might have surfaced. Anything you are told in confidence during a Reiki session should absolutely stay in between you and your client, regardless of whether he is a close friend or a stranger. The client is inclined to open up more after the treatment than originally intended, and must then be able to trust the practitioner completely. If you lack required education do not counsel your client or act as a psychologist during these conversations! What most people need in a sensitive situation is somebody who is able to listen and who shows compassion and understanding. Lend your ear during this time, listen patiently, and allow yourself the beauty of experiencing how well the client is able to structure any problems and to find answers to his own questions while talking in this accepting space.

It is very common that the client falls asleep during the treatment. Sleeping might be a passive escape from oneself and previous experiences, but the client still receives full benefit from the Reiki. Let the client sleep until it is time to turn over or until you are finishing off the treatment. It is normally easier to stay awake after a few treatments, but most clients relax so deeply they may appear to be asleep. The belly might rumble, which is the physical evidence of the body resolving some deep-seated emotions. Small muscles in the face, arms and legs may twitch or jerk when releasing suppressed tensions. At times the client may start to cry. Keep tissues handy for these occasions. In rare cases the client may go into regression, i.e., a previously suppressed and painful memory surfaces and the client reacts with loud crying and/or screaming. Reiki initiated this process, but Reiki also helps the client to resolve the painful event in a harmonious way. *Always continue to give Reiki whatever the reactions!* Reiki nurture and heals, and afterwards the client will experience an enormous relief.

Reiki is a very gentle technique that makes us aware and remember without bringing forth more than we are able to handle at that moment. The client will never be overwhelmed by his past and more so, the person you treat will not react in a stronger way than what you as a practitioner will be able to manage. In other words, you never have to worry about treating a client whose problems are larger than you or he can handle. That will not happen.

The client may experience certain bodily reactions and discomfort the first few days after the initial treatments. The most common counteractions are light headache, nausea and diarrhea. This is the body's natural way of discharging toxins accumulated over the years. Mood swings may occur as suppressed emotions are released. Physical discomfort and pains that have been long gone may sometimes reappear and linger for a short while.

Normally, receiving treatments does not create as strong a healing crisis as having Reiki activated in the body system during a seminar. The Reiki attunements cause a speed up of the body's energy vibrations. In order for the body to regain balance in its new state it might need to go through a more powerful cleansing. Also when giving someone a Reiki treatment for the first time a clean-out of stored waste products and emotions is initiated, but normally not as strong. The client may experience increased pain or worse symptoms before starting to feel better. Do not pay too much attention to what discomfort might arise while discussing the effects of the treatment. The client's own expectations may then cause more discomfort than need be, and he might feel worse than necessary. It is important, however, to make the client perfectly aware of this possible healing crisis in order to understand and embrace the reactions that might occur.

Most of the discomfort will disappear after the second treatment. Therefore, it is important that the client returns as soon as possible to continue being treated, preferably the following day. If you give three consecutive treatments close to one another, the time and intensity of any discomfort is lessened. Every person will experience Reiki differently. On some occasions the emotional clean-out in particular may be delayed by several treatments. Remember also that many people do not experience any healing crisis at all.

An energy exchange between you and the client sets up the best opportunity for a good healing climate. Both you and your time will be more appreciated, and you will achieve optimal results from the treatments. Money is one of the energies that is used in order to trade other energies, for instance a treatment, but services in the form of a barter system can also be traded. (Within the family there is an ongoing energy exchange occurring, and you obviously do not have to worry about charging your family members.)

To give something in exchange for a treatment feels right to most people. There are few who like to build up a debt account to somebody else. If you do not accept payment in some way or other from your clients they might be uncomfortable coming back since they feel in debt but are not allowed to repay. It is also true that many people take a subconscious but determined decision to get well by actively contributing to their own recovery by giving something in return. You will also feel better when others appreciate the time you give them.

It may be difficult at first, but it is important to recognize that you and your time has a value, and charging for your treatments is very good for your sense of self-worth.

Use the treatments to develop your intuition. Learn to "listen" to your hands. Become aware of how different people draw different amounts of energy, and how different parts of the same body also can feel different. It is quite common that the client experiences your hands in one way, while your feeling is totally different. For instance, the person you are treating may feel your hands as very warm, while you experience coldness in the very same area. With some practice you will intuitively know what illnesses, pains and problems the client suffers from. While learning to trust your intuition you may check with the client to find out if your assumptions are right. However, *never* frighten anybody by saying that you think you have discovered a serious disease. You can be wrong! If you are absolutely sure, and fully capable of tuning in to your intuition, tell the client that you can feel an imbalance in the energies around the particular area or organ that you suspect. You may carefully advise the client to have a health checkup. Never make any diagnoses! If you do not have the appropriate education, you have no right to assume the role of a physician. Besides, it is absolutely unnecessary to make any diagnoses since Reiki is automatically drawn to the areas needed, regardless of whether you know where that would be or not. So again, keep your ego out of the treatment.

Some practitioners have an intuitive ability to feel the client's pain in their own body, exactly in the areas where the client has problems, pain or illnesses. This phenomenon is quite natural, and is a normal expression of the psychic ability of particularly sensitive individuals. Do not become afraid if this would happen to you. Just allow the energy to flow freely, and visualize yourself surrounded by light. The pain or discomfort you feel will disappear as soon as you lift your hands from the client's body or soon thereafter. Practitioners who feel the client's pain in this way develop their intuition by letting these feelings guide their hands to the right position on the body.

Some practitioners use their inner vision to "see" where the client has a problem, and where the hands should be placed in order to achieve the best result. Other practitioners have an inner knowing of where to place their hands, while others again feel the "pull" of energy drawn by the client's body when placing their hands on areas requiring extra Reiki. It is quite common that the practitioner becomes warm and might start sweating during the treatment due to the energy flowing through his body. In the beginning you may feel nothing at all, neither from your hands nor intuitively, but the more you use your Reiki, both on yourself and others, the more you will develop your intuition and the sensitivity of your hands.

Everyone who has attended a First Degree Reiki Seminar, and received the four attunements, has the same energy flow in their hands. The same energy frequency is activated in everybody, but each one will experience the feeling of Reiki completely differently, depending on how experienced they are in working with subtle energies. Each individual has their own interpretation of the feelings of Reiki, and the sensation in the hands can vary enormously. It is very common for the hands to feel warm, or in some cases extremely hot, while some again experience coldness, tingling, prickles, tickles, numbness, an itch in the palm of their hands, or absolutely nothing at all. None of this is right or wrong. Reiki is always the same. It is the interpretation or the sensation of Reiki that varies, depending on our background and ability to comprehend.

During the Reiki treatment it is important that you focus on your client. This way the treatment becomes more exciting since you will rapidly learn to distinguish between different sensations in your hands when resting on different parts of the body. You will also find that every person you treat feels different from the others. The strength of the treatment is mainly determined by your focus. You do not have to fully concentrate on Reiki, but avoid letting your thoughts drift to your own problems and worries as that is not fair to the client who on a subtle level might be affected by your mood. If you have committed yourself to do the treatment, you have to be present with more than just a physical body.

The more of yourself you put into a project, the more you and everybody involved will get out of it. If you listlessly sit by the client in boredom, you have somehow missed the purpose of Reiki and might just as well not give the treatment. It is not ethically right to offer your help to someone if you are unable to live up to your promise on an energetic level. Once you have initiated the treatment it should always be carried out on the client's terms, but whether to give a treatment or not in the first place—that is your decision! If you do not have the time or the inclination at that particular moment, you should not give the treatment at all.

CHILDREN AND REIKI

Small children do not have the same need for full treatments as adults do. They have not yet protected themselves with subtle armor or built up massive blockages in their bodies. The energy will therefore flow more freely and the treatments can be shortened. Young children do not have the same patience as adults or older children, and they should never be forced to receive treatments; that would only create resistance and then it might be difficult to give them any Reiki at all. Children have small bodies and the hands of an adult easily cover most of a child's torso therefore fewer positions can be used. Twenty to thirty minutes of Reiki is often sufficient, but the length of the treatment always depends on how long the child wants to be still. Do not make a big fuss about the treatments as that might create resistance. If the child does not want to lie down for the treatment, you may try giving Reiki when you are sitting together doing other things. Place your hands in a comfortable position on the child when he is on your lap, or next to you on the couch watching TV. The child does not even have to know what you are doing. Be relaxed! You do not have to stick to the adult recommendations such as being quiet and still during the treatment. Give the child the freedom he needs.

Some children love to receive Reiki and they ask for their treatment every day. Others do not want Reiki at all or only during times when they have hurt themselves or are sick. Reiki is an outstanding pain-relief with regards to bruises, bumps, wasp's stings, cuts, minor burns and other injuries children are often subject to, but remember to always see a physician if the injury seems serious. You can give Reiki on the way to the doctor, in the waiting room and afterwards.

Children are very intuitive, and when sick they often have the ability to sense the importance of Reiki. They are usually willing to receive more frequent treatments than healthy and active children. In sick children who receive Reiki treatments the results can be astonishing.

Hyperactive children do not usually want to receive any Reiki, and it can be difficult to give them treatments since they are unable to be still for more than a few minutes at the time. One way to overcome this problem is to give them Reiki when they are asleep. You can quietly go into the bedroom and place your hands anywhere on the child's body without waking her. Stay there for twenty or so minutes. After receiving Reiki this way for some time the child may calm down and might even start to ask for treatments.

Some children become so interested in Reiki they want to learn it for themselves. There are Reiki Masters who give short seminars for children. Children are given the four attunements and the ability to use Reiki remains for the rest of their lives. Personally I give seminars to children between five and twelve years of age, since it is important that they are old enough to decide for themselves whether they want Reiki or not.

I never accept children who do not want to participate, regardless of their parents' opinion. Children should be respected as individuals with free will and identity. Before I agree to the child being attuned I make sure that at least one of the parents or guardians also have Reiki, to be able to guide the child and answer questions that later might arise.

During the hormonal changes of pre-puberty and the following emotional turbulence children begin to block up and will require longer treatments. At this age it is appropriate to apply the full one hour treatments. The hormonal changes are also the reason why teenagers cannot attend the children's seminar. Just like adults, they will need more space in between the four attunements than what is permitted during the shorter children's seminar.

GROUP REIKI

Two energy frequencies of the same kind that meet become more than their sum total, and the energy is virtually squared. As a general rule you can say that when two people come together to give Reiki their energy is squared, and instead of one hour of Reiki the client receives 2 x 2 = 4 hours worth of Reiki. ($2^2 = 4$) The two practitioners working together give four minutes worth of Reiki for each minute of treatment. When three people give Reiki at the same time the energies are also squared so that the worth of Reiki per minute is 3 x 3 = 9 minutes. ($3^2 = 9$) The squared energy of four people gives 4 x 4 = 16 minutes worth of Reiki per minute and so on. ($4^2 = 16, 5^2 = 25, 6^2 = 36...$)

It is possible to benefit from this phenomenon by meeting in a group and giving each other short but very powerful treatments. Even ten minutes of Reiki can give a substantial supply of energy when several persons contribute their Reiki energy. The way to do this is simple. One person lies down on the treatment table. One person sits at the top end and treats the head, and one sits at the bottom end to treat the feet. The rest of the group gather around the table and place their hands on the torso and legs. The group rotates one step after each treatment so that everybody gets to place their hands in different positions. This is a good opportunity to develop the feeling of sensations in the hands.

Ask the client before the group treatment starts whether he has got any particular problems or pains where he would like to have somebody's hands placed. Since the person receiving the treatment also has Reiki he can contribute by comfortably placing his hands on his own body. The treatment normally takes ten minutes. The client turns onto his stomach after half the time and the back is treated in the same way during the last five minutes. The person at the head is the timekeeper and tells everybody when it is time to switch.

As an example: if six people decide to meet and give each other ten minutes of Reiki per person, each one will receive 6 x 6 = 36 x 10 = 360 minutes worth of Reiki. ($6^2 = 36, 36 x 10 = 360$) This is roughly 6 hours of Reiki, in ten minutes! Five people give the treatment, but the sixth person also counts since he treats himself while receiving the treatment by placing his hands on his own body.

A group Reiki session normally lasts about one and a half to two hours, depending on the number of people present. It is important to arrive on time and to stay until everybody has had their share. Group Reiki does not only mean to receive but also to give of oneself to others. If everybody arrives towards the end just to receive their own treatment, there would be no group Reiki at all.

Group Reiki differs from ordinary treatments, as they are pretty free and without particular recommendations. The social part is just as important as giving and receiving Reiki. It is therefore okay to talk during the treatments. The meeting also gives an opportunity to discuss, laugh and exchange experiences. A ten to fifteen minute treatment is not long enough to relax deeply, but the person receiving Reiki should of course try to keep quiet and enjoy the nurturing energy. Some groups still choose to give the treatments in silence since this gives the client a more tranquil experience. They usually finish the meeting off with tea and coffee and do their talking then.

A group can consist of anything from three to ten or more people. The more people at the same table, the longer time the treatment of the whole group will take. It might therefore be worthwhile to split a larger group in two. A healthy person is not able to draw energy from more than what is given by about five to six people at the same time, while a very sick person draws the squared energy from many more. In a large group of healthy individuals this means that the Reiki energy does not flow with full strength from the people giving the treatment, since the client will not draw more than the body needs. This mechanism works like a natural fuse in the system, and makes it impossible to over-treat somebody with Reiki.

An established Reiki group may meet every week, or every second week, but more common is maybe once a month. Joining a Reiki group has many advantages. There is always someone to call if you need to talk, there is often a good atmosphere at the meetings, and the subjects of conversation are many and varied. You can learn a lot from your Reiki friends, and many groups continue to meet outside of the actual Reiki event. They may attend other seminars and lectures together, or meet just for a chat. Starting a Reiki group is an excellent way of making friends for life, as well as regularly receiving a substantial energy boost.

MARATHON REIKI

Some Reiki groups have mutual agreements to help each other if one of them would get sick. If this happens the group will do a marathon Reiki. Marathon Reiki is a way of helping a seriously ill person by gathering the group together to give the sick person Reiki for a substantial amount of time. The one treated might be someone from the group or a close friend or relative. The group decides on a particular time, maybe two or three hours on a Saturday or Sunday afternoon when most people are free. The sick person lays on the treatment table to receive Reiki during the whole event, while the people in the group come and go as their time and means allow. Some people may stay for the whole time, while others might stop by for half an hour or an hour. Whatever one is able to offer at a time like this is a beautiful gift towards the benefit and health of another.

Giving of oneself to a fellow human being who is seriously ill is very fulfilling. It is also reassuring to know that you have a group behind you that will support you would it become necessary. The extended treatment session, given by many people together, may provide just that extra kick needed to help somebody recover from a serious illness. On other occasions marathon Reiki has assisted people by offering pain-relief, and/or a means to better handle the situation before dying.

WHEN REIKI APPEARS NOT TO WORK

I sometimes get the question: why does Reiki not work? The person suffering from a certain problem does not appear to get any better, in spite of repeated Reiki treatments.

When the ailment or problem is minor, but the client does not seem to respond to the treatment, it is often because a more severe imbalance in the body is drawing the energy. Reiki heals by priority. That means Reiki is attracted to the most severe imbalances first. These imbalances may be related to problems or ailments in the body that have not yet been detected. Reiki is automatically attracted to these areas, regardless of whether we try to direct the energy to other areas of the body or not.

Reiki goes far beyond our limited ego. We have nothing to do with the healing that takes place, all we do is temporarily lend our hands to somebody else during the treatment. It is the Reiki energy that supplies the intelligence, and creates the harmony required in order for the body to heal itself more effectively. We do not know what is going on inside the body and where Reiki is drawn. If there is no improvement in the area we are treating it is easy to assume the energy has simply been attracted to other more important locations in the body.

In some cases we know that we are treating a very serious disease and it is highly improbable that something else in the body can be in greater need. Why is it then that the Reiki treatments do not seem to help in these cases?

Sometimes the decay of the body has simply gone too far. No matter how much Reiki is given, it never seems to catch up with the disease and turn the process around. These times we are simply involved in the natural cycle of life and death. The body is born, it lives, and after a while it is worn out and dies. When we have accomplished what we came here to do, regardless of age, it is time to continue the journey in other dimensions. Reiki will never stop or interfere in that process. That would be the same as interfering with Universal Law. Instead, Reiki helps us relieve pain and fears, and prepares us for the journey.

Karma is another reason why Reiki sometimes, on a superficial level, does not seem to have any greater effect. Karma means cause and effect, i.e., what goes around comes around, or as you sow shall you reap. This should not be literally translated into only the number of years that constitute a lifetime. When looking at Karma we have to see the bigger picture where we all have a function in infinite time. We have acted and reacted in lifetime after lifetime. In some cases with mercy and compassion, in others with hatred and cruelty. Everything we do creates a counter-effect, just like in physics.

The period between the cause, our action, and the effect that our action has implacably caused, can be enormous according to our concept of time. Despite this, at some point there will be a time when we will have to face and work through the Karma we once created. Karma is not a punishment, it is just a repayment or re-balancing of the energies we once emitted. Some of these payments will lead to positive changes in our life while others will provide difficulties, accidents and diseases to overcome. The Karma we are working through will result in increased understanding, insight, development, courage and compassion.

Reiki will not protect us from serious Karmic debts that need to be settled, but it might help in improving the situation. We might not have to suffer as much pain, or be stuck in the process for as long as we would without Reiki. Reiki always works, but it might not always work in the way we in our limited understanding would like it to.

Another reason for an illness to persist might be the own blocked self. Maybe we are not yet ready to let go of the illness. Perhaps it gives us advantages that we subconsciously would like to keep. Maybe we do not want to see the necessity of changing our lifestyle in order to get well. A disease occurs when we have failed in our communication with our body. The body's last resort to make us listen is to fall ill. If we refuse to change, the situation might even go as far as to the death of the physical body. Unfortunately this occurs far too often, despite the intricate protection system of symptoms and diseases developing in our body to show us we are treating it wrongly. In some very serious cases the reason for not healing might be Soul choosing to leave a stagnated situation where It sees no potential for further development.

Reiki aids our growth and development. It expands our awareness, and increases the ability to listen to the body and its needs. It will then become easier to understand if we are living a disharmonious life in some way or other. That insight can help us change our situation, and in doing so the need for the disease will disappear.

Still, one of the most common reasons as to why Reiki does not always seem to work is probably this: With the help of Reiki, the possibility of unfoldment and inner growth becomes immensely enhanced—that is *if* we use our Reiki. If we take advantage of Reiki it becomes easier to see what we can change about ourselves, and how we can choose another direction, in order to avoid the necessity of disease. If we do not use the opportunity for health that Reiki offers, or only apply it sporadically, it will obviously not have that effect.

Reiki is an aid. It is a tool to help us feel better. Reiki supplies energy to the body, it speeds-up cell rejuvenation and tissue repairs, it enhances the natural healing process of the body, etc. In order for this tool to work it must be used. A nail does not jump into the wall by itself. We have to use a tool—the hammer—to put the nail into the wall by our own effort, using the hammer as an aid. Look at Reiki the same way. If we do not use Reiki regularly, in the daily one hour treatment, we reduce our chances of optimal well-being. We are denying ourselves the opportunity to reach the maximum potential of vitality, health and harmony.

It is not easy to predict how the body will react when treating ourselves or others with Reiki. We are all individuals with different root causes to our problems and illnesses. Every person will have a unique reaction and course of a disease, even when the illness appears to be the same on the surface. I do not want you to be fanatical with your Reiki. I just want you to understand the value of the gift you have been given. My hope is that this book will give you a better insight into the works of Reiki, and how you easily can use the advantages of Reiki in order to achieve the best and quickest improvements in your own life.

SEVEN

OTHER TREATMENTS

From the moment Reiki is activated in the body the energy radiates from the hands at the slightest touch of any living being. All organic matter is alive and is therefore positively affected by the Reiki you give. Through regular Reiki treatments you can create great improvements and healing in both animals and plants. All matter consists of vibrating fields of energy, therefore the scope of Reiki is much larger than you might initially think.

TREATING ANIMALS

Most animals love to receive Reiki treatments. Furthermore, animals are in much better harmony with their bodies and their needs than man, and they often know how much Reiki is needed for different ailments. When the animal has had enough it simply shrugs the hands off its body or walks away. The normal treatment time for a healthy animal would be about twenty minutes. This does not mean you have to stop giving Reiki after this time if the animal is still and seems to enjoy the touch and closeness. You can never give too much Reiki, neither to animals nor humans.

The size of the animal has no importance to the length of the treatment. A horse or a kitten, both take as long to treat. The Reiki energy flows faster and easier through the body of an animal than through the body of a human. Animals are normally not as blocked as human beings, even if some sensitive pets can adopt the neuroses of their owner and become nervous themselves. In those cases it is often worthwhile to treat the owner as well. Generally animals have a freer and stronger energy field than humans, and they normally require much shorter treatments. When giving Reiki to a small animal in your lap, it often wriggles into the perfect position for the hands to fall in the place where the Reiki is most needed.

Cats in particular are very sensitive to energies and sometimes perceive Reiki as too strong. Initially the animal may become frightened by the tangible energy Reiki emits. It might need some time to get used to the energy and should naturally never be forced to receive a treatment. Cats often need a day or two to get used to its "new" owner after he or she has had Reiki activated. The cat reacts when sensing the massive extension and changes in the aura caused by the attunements. Cats are curious animals and sometimes they will cautiously sniff the hands of their owner in wonder, trying to figure out what new and different energy is brought home. The cat might even sniff around the entire body of its owner before contentedly lying down on top of the hands to take part of the energy.

Some animals only want to receive Reiki if they have hurt themselves or are ill. Then they might voluntarily come for a treatment. Animals are individuals just like humans, and we have to allow the same freedom to them as we would want for ourselves. We can never force ourselves upon an animal that does not want to sit still to receive Reiki. We can only accept their choice, whatever that might be.

TREATING PLANTS

Plants of all kinds: trees, bushes, potted plants, garden plants, etc. flourish with the help of Reiki. The best way of giving Reiki to plants is by holding your hands around or close to the root system, since that is where the plant takes in the nourishment. Treat the plant for about twenty minutes. Sick and weak plants can be given more frequent and longer treatments. Potted plants are easy to treat. You simply hold your hands around the pot and let the energy flow into the plant. The energy can pass through plastic, ceramics and other pot materials without any problems. Trees, bushes and other garden plants require a bit more effort since the result will be best if you place your hands close to the root system or at the bottom of the trunk. An easier alternative for the vegetable garden is to give ten minutes of Reiki to the seed bag before planting the seeds. This extra supply of Reiki energy enhances the inherent Life Force of the seed and provides faster growth, and bigger, healthier flowers and vegetables.

If you have had Reiki activated in your hands you might find it interesting to experiment with different seeds from the same bag. You can, for instance, give Reiki to half of the seeds and leave the rest untouched. Keep track of which portion is which and see how much faster the seeds receiving Reiki will grow. Remember not to touch the control group, i.e. the seeds that are not supposed to be given Reiki. One of my Reiki students planted a handful of sunflower seeds. The entire process took approximately ten minutes. The flowers growing from the seeds that had been in her hand the longest grew twice as fast as the seeds she planted first and which had not received as much Reiki. The row of sunflowers grew up in an increasing scale, with the largest and longest flowers at the end of the row.

You can do other interesting experiments with sprouts, such as alfalfa, lentils or mung beans. Give Reiki to one part of the seeds and keep a control group that does not receive Reiki. Treat the experiment sprouts daily for twenty minutes and you will soon see the difference between them and the sprouts that do not get Reiki. Remember that nature is unpredictable and that your results may vary accordingly.

Vegetables keep their elasticity and vigor better with the help of Reiki. As an experiment you may cut a tomato or some other vegetable or fruit in two halves. Keep the two halves in the same environment, but separated by at least fifty centimeters. Select one of the halves and give it daily Reiki treatments. I have followed such a tomato experiment for over four years. A fresh, healthy tomato was cut in two, each half placed in separate glass jars with lids. One of the halves received Reiki every day for four weeks through the jar. Thereafter the application of Reiki was limited to a couple of treatments a month. The second tomato half was left without receiving any Reiki. After six weeks the untreated half was decomposed to a fermented juicy mess, covered with mold. The tomato half receiving Reiki was still keeping its shape after four years! Except a dried surface, faded color, and some liquid in the bottom of the jar, it still looked like a relatively healthy half tomato.

These types of experiments can be both fun and exciting, at the same time as it helps you see that your Reiki works, gives you better self-confidence, and makes you more accustomed to Reiki. It should be added that the tomato experiment that I followed for four years was unusually successful. It is more common that the fruit or vegetable treated with Reiki lasts a few days, weeks or months longer than the untreated control group or control half.

An alternative to crawling around in your garden applying Reiki to each vegetable is giving five to ten minutes of Reiki to the watering-can before watering. This way the water is charged with energy and while watering, your plants also receive an extra energy kick. Even if the strength cannot be compared to a proper Reiki treatment it is a good alternative if you have lots of flowers and vegetables to care for.

FOOD, DRINK AND CIGARETTES

Giving Reiki does not remove toxins and residues from chemical substances that might remain in the food, but you will help the body digest the meal by providing a little Reiki before you eat. The body will be able to absorb more of the vitamins, minerals and nutrients in the food. Giving a few minutes of Reiki to the food when eating out is also a good idea. It is quite common that the environment in the restaurant kitchen is stressed and perhaps filled with anger and irritation. This stress, in combination with other unhealthy emotional energies, is stored in the food when cooked. After eating such a meal we might feel bloated, and our stomachs rumble when trying to digest the congested emotions we just ate. A couple of minutes of Reiki before eating will balance the negative energies that might have been stored in the food and we will feel better after the meal. It is worthwhile to give your food at home a quick Reiki treatment too, in order to help the body absorb the nutrients it receives more efficiently.

The same goes for different kinds of drinks. Most of us know that coffee and tea are no health drinks, but we still want to enjoy them from time to time. Giving Reiki by holding your hands around the cup will help the liver to break down caffeine, tannin and other less healthy products that might be found in the drink.

Giving Reiki to what we eat and drink does not mean that unhealthy drinks and junk food are okay. Instead, using Reiki means we acquire a better harmony with our body and our needs. A natural consequence is often that the desire for unhealthy products decreases. The consumption of alcohol has also been seen to decrease in the same way. Even people who only drink socially and not much at all seem to lessen their alcohol consumption after starting to use Reiki regularly. In some cases the body reacts so strongly to alcohol that it becomes difficult to drink even smaller quantities. The body's reactions always show us its weak spots and is thereby helping us abstain from substances that are particularly harmful. Each individual reacts differently and to achieve better health we must learn to listen to, and follow, the signals from our own bodies.

Smoking is another area where Reiki might help. It is easier for a person who is using Reiki on a regular basis to stop smoking than for somebody who does not have Reiki. The body is gradually balanced by the energy, and the need for harmful and addictive products lessen. The change can be immediate or take its time. Sometimes the process may take several years depending on how seriously the body is affected by the smoking. Different individuals are affected to different extents. Sometimes Reiki prioritizes other areas in the body before the smoking issue is attended.

INANIMATE OBJECTS

Reiki has the ability to harmonize and balance the energies in all organic matter. What might be more surprising is Reiki's capacity to affect inanimate objects. I have been told numerous stories about discharged car batteries being sufficiently charged by Reiki to actually start the engine. That batteries contain organic matter in the form of carbon might be one explanation why they are affected by Reiki. Theoretically it is quite impossible that inanimate objects would react to Reiki, especially with the speed with which they actually do. I will not discuss how and why inanimate objects are influenced by Reiki, but I would like to mention a few episodes that I have come in contact with, particularly through my Reiki students.

It is usually an easy task to open frozen car locks and petrol caps by giving a couple of minutes of Reiki. One of my friends in New Zealand repaired her washing-machine by giving it Reiki. Some other broken objects that have been mended with the aid of Reiki are a stove, CD-players, radios, tape-recorders, loud-speakers, TVs, video games, remote controls, cellular phones and kettles, among many other things. Electrical appliances seem to be high on my students list for Reiki treatments.

Personally I think there is no harm in trying Reiki when something breaks down in the house. There is nothing to lose, and at more times than can be attributed to chance the broken object starts to work again and the money on repair is saved.

As you can see, the field of application extends far beyond what we initially might associate with Reiki. This makes the energy even more exciting and interesting to work with. The experiments can be many and creative. The technique for Reiki always remains the same: a simple touch, allowing the energy to flow freely into damaged or imbalanced areas, easily, naturally and without side-effects.

EIGHT

Associations and Training

*H*awayo Takata brought the Usui System of Reiki from Japan via Hawaii to the USA and Canada. Reiki had already begun to spread outside the borders of North America at her death in 1980. Starting at 1970 Takata trained twenty-two new Reiki Masters before she died. Her aim was for them to continue to spread the technique of Reiki throughout the world.

The Reiki training and the content of the seminars has since branched out in different directions and opinions as to what Reiki is and how it should be taught, mainly due to different individual's beliefs and opinions. Because of this the set up of the seminars may differ quite substantially between different Reiki Masters and associations. The standard and quality, both of the Master and the seminars, may also vary from not so good to excellent. In spite of the great variations between different Reiki Masters, everyone attending a seminar receives the same Reiki energy in their hands. Providing of course that the attunements are correctly performed! This cannot always be guaranteed with regards to Reiki Masters who have been through a crash course where quantity has taken precedence over quality. It is important to understand that the attunement techniques have to be followed correctly in order for Reiki to be *permanently* activated in a person's hands and body systems.

Associations
Today there is no person or association that is holding the overall responsibility, and that governs the standard of the training of all the Reiki

Masters throughout the world. Instead, many different Reiki associations have been founded over the years. As early as in 1979, Hawayo Takata and one of her students, Barbara Webber Ray, founded the first Reiki association which was given the name A.R.A. (The American Reiki Association). A.R.A. was renamed A.I.R.A. (The American International Reiki Association) after Takata's death. Barbara Webber Ray became the new president. Takata's Grand-daughter, Phyllis Lei Furumoto, founded a new association called the Reiki Alliance in 1981. Some of the twenty-two Reiki Masters trained by Takata joined the new association but most remained independent. The two associations differ in their methods of teaching Reiki, but the traditional attunement process is the same.

THE REIKI ALLIANCE

The Reiki Alliance has tried to maintain Reiki the way it was taught by Mikao Usui, and the seminars held by the members of the association are often very practical. The Reiki Alliance has the largest number of members of the existing associations and is probably, because of this, the most well-known. Previously the Reiki Alliance did not have any stated requirements for the training of Reiki Masters, and the structure of the seminars tends to vary substantially between different Reiki Masters within the association. Certain regulations have been introduced but there have been some problems in the members accepting and adopting the new changes and ideas. Due to this, the Reiki Alliance is an association with great variations in its member's standard of training and quality of seminars. The Reiki Alliance stresses the spirituality of Reiki, and a religious touch might be added to the teaching. Reiki, however, does not belong to any following, and any attempt to make it so is outside of its scope.

The Reiki Alliance is closely linked to the person of Phyllis Lei Furumoto, claiming that she is the leading Reiki Grand Master of the world. However, Hawayo Takata did not officially designate any of the Reiki Masters trained by her as her particular successor. Phyllis Lei Furumoto renounced her membership of the Reiki Alliance in July of 1992. For several years she worked independently before she once again reclaimed her position with the Reiki Alliance. Since 1997 Phyllis

Lei Furumoto has been working hard to patent the Usui System of Reiki in several countries. This might seem a bit odd since the technique of Reiki has spread all over the world, is used by millions of people, and is taught by thousands of Reiki Masters from many different associations and independent sources.

A.I.R.A—THE RADIANCE TECHNIQUE

A.I.R.A., which is now called T.R.T. (The Radiance Technique) has spent much time and money researching Reiki. Many new facts have surfaced, and both the seminars and the training of Masters has developed dramatically. On the whole it is T.R.T. that has provided most of the scientific knowledge about Reiki that we have today. The Radiance Technique is strict in their requirements on education, and has set regulations for what is to be taught in the different degrees and what the Master Training should contain. The members are generally holding a high standard. In order to stress the difference in structure and training of their members in comparison to other Reiki Masters, A.I.R.A. changed their name to The Radiance Technique. They stress the scientific side of Reiki. T.R.T. only accepts Reiki Masters who have been trained by their own members, and it is impossible to enter in any other way. The Radiance Technique is a smaller association active mainly in the USA. There are a few members found in Europe and other parts of the world. Today T.R.T. refuses any association with the name Reiki, stating they teach a different technique all together. The attunement process of Reiki, however, remains the same.

INDEPENDENT REIKI MASTERS

Independent Reiki Masters follow, in their seminar curriculum and training of new Masters, either the Reiki Alliance, T.R.T. or any of the new associations that have been established, depending on which Master influenced their training. The standard of an independent Reiki Master's seminars therefore varies greatly, and depends entirely on the Master Teacher who performed their training.

THE REIKI NETWORK

Many new associations have been established throughout the world in the last couple of decades. The Reiki Network was founded by John and Esther Veltheim in 1990. The objectives of the association are to spread the use of Reiki all over the world, maintain a high standard of teaching, and to keep up a fellowship and networking between affiliated Reiki Masters. Today the Reiki Network is teaching in many countries all over the world in a number of different languages.

The Reiki Network is a politically independent association with a clearly defined minimum standard of education that has to be met by the Reiki Masters applying for membership. The Reiki Network requires their members to go through a training program, following a set manual, in order to acquire a sound understanding of Reiki and its benefits. When teaching seminars the members must meet at least these set minimum requirements. Though the curriculum must be followed the members are also encouraged to maintain their personal touch and to adjust their seminars to cultural needs.

A certain minimum amount of information must be taught at each degree in order for the Reiki Master's membership to be approved. It is not possible to become a member unless the Master has gone through the approved education. Any Reiki Master, regardless of background, can become a member as soon as he or she can adequately show that he/she meets the specified minimum requirements. Additional training for Reiki Masters who wish to apply for membership can be arranged. The education is standardized, and The Reiki Network guarantees that every member maintains a high standard of lecturing and a uniformity in the distributed information. This makes it possible for a student to change Reiki Masters within the Reiki Network and still be able to follow the seminar program. Hence, it is possible to do the First Degree with one Reiki Master but choose to do the Second Degree with another Master within the association. A student who has not done the First Degree with a Network Master, but who wishes to do the Second Degree with a member, is recommended to first monitor the First Degree. It may be difficult to benefit from the extensive material in the following degrees without first repeating the First Degree seminar to receive all the basic information given by the Network Master.

The Reiki Network was founded so that individuals wanting to learn Reiki would have the opportunity to choose a Reiki Master with a guaranteed thorough education, and be sure to attend a seminar of high quality. Further, the association is there for the affiliated Reiki Masters to utilize the networking idea of recommending each other to interested students in places outside of their own teaching areas. The referred students can be assured that these Masters have a seminar program and a training that equals their own Master's. The number of Reiki Masters world wide, who are members of the Reiki Network, is steadily increasing.

The Reiki Network is regularly sending out a newsletter with articles and contemporary information in order to keep its members up to date with new development and knowledge. The association presents Reiki as an energy science based on modern physics and metaphysics alike.

TRAINING

The different opinions about Reiki and how it should be taught have led to the development of different ways of training and how to give seminars. The Reiki Alliance has kept the three original degrees of Reiki, while The Radiance Technique has developed several new degrees and has a total of ten levels in their training. Today the most common is probably that Reiki is taught in five degrees. This latter procedure has been accepted by the Reiki Network, most independent Reiki Masters and some members of the Reiki Alliance.

These five levels consist of: the First Degree, the Second Degree, the Third Degree or 3A—for personal development, the Reiki Master Degree, and Reiki Master Teacher or Grand Master Degree. The Reiki Alliance does not recognize the 3A Degree. They take their students directly from the Second Degree to the Master training. This is proven to be a big and many times very difficult step in a person's development. It also limits the number of students who wish to take their personal growth as far as possible using Reiki.

THE FIRST DEGREE

The First Degree of Reiki is by far the most important step for anybody. In this seminar the Reiki is activated in the body systems and will remain in the person for the rest of their life. Reiki works as a preventive health-care program, helping to accelerate the body's own healing process, enhancing personal development and expanding awareness, creating increased inner understanding, etc. Life will start to change in many positive ways after participating in the First Degree seminar, especially for the participants who choose to use their Reiki on a regular basis. In this seminar the students learn what Reiki is, how it works, and how to use the technique on themselves and others in order to achieve the best results. The students learn to give Reiki by passively placing their hands on the body allowing the energy to flow freely to any areas of imbalance. Reiki is a holistic therapy that creates harmony on all levels: physically, emotionally, mentally and spiritually. Correctly used Reiki brings joy, harmony, insight, development and improved physical health in everyone who receives the four attunements and then continues to use the technique regularly.

The length of the seminar should include two full days, at least ten but rather twelve to fourteen hours. This will allow appropriate time for lecturing, practical hands-on exercises and attunements. The First Degree seminar is complete in itself. There is no need for additional seminars after Reiki has been activated in the body systems. This is important to understand when receiving Reiki, in case you might be told you are only half-way through after your First Degree. The subsequent seminars are for practitioners and for those who are keen to develop their Reiki in learning more advanced and exciting techniques, but remember that the First Degree is complete in itself, even if there are additional techniques to be learned by an active and inquisitive student. For these people it is a natural step to go on to the next level, the Second Degree.

THE SECOND DEGREE OR THE PRACTITIONERS DEGREE

The Second Degree teaches different advanced techniques of how to guide the Reiki energy to particular areas or concepts you might want to work with. Three symbols or energy formulas are taught which, when correctly used, will rearrange and change other patterns of energy into greater harmony and balance. One might work on changing the physical energies of the body towards better health, but one may as well be working on subtle energies like an unhappy situation or relationship, a particular belief system or conditioning, a specific fear, phobia or addiction, or the influence of a difficult childhood and upbringing, just to mention a few of the areas that can be improved by using the techniques from the Second Degree.

Reiki is an unpolarized energy that vibrates many times faster than the speed of light. The human being's conception of time and space follows the physical laws of our universe. Energies outside of this physical dimension have other time conditions and another conception of space. Since Reiki moves beyond our known dimension, the energy does not behave in the same way as we are used to in our physical world. Reiki has a completely different ability of instantaneously moving between various events beyond our known time/space reality. During the entire 20th century scientists have been fascinated by the rapidly moving frequencies existing outside of our limited consciousness. These energies move and work totally independently of known physical laws and understanding. Reiki is one of these unexplored energies of the quantum physics, and therefore Reiki also has the ability to instantaneously and effortlessly move through time and space.

The main reason why many people choose to go on to the Second Degree is because they want to learn how to send absentee Reiki treatments. The sender might, for example, be sitting in the United States sending Reiki to Australia, Sweden or anywhere else in the world, and the treatment is instantaneously received by the recipient. The distance loses its meaning as Reiki vibrates at a frequency beyond the speed of light. Further advantages is that it only takes fifteen minutes to send a complete one hour treatment, and that it is possible to send Reiki to several people at the same time. The ability to send Reiki will help reduce the feelings of powerlessness and anxiety that can be experienced when our loved ones are ill or have other problems but are too far away to be reached personally. A Reiki practitioner using the Second Degree techniques can effectively help another person even when he or she resides in another place, city or country.

Many people who have sick relatives living far away choose to take the next level of Reiki solely to help these individuals, but the Second Degree has much more to offer than that. The students will for instance learn how to protect themselves, others, and their belongings. They learn how to give themselves a short but very powerful Reiki treatment. They are taught a specific and very effective Chakra treatment. The participants also learn how to strengthen their affirmations, thereby accelerating the entire process, i.e. achieving quicker and more tangible results.

The Second Degree also includes techniques to create harmony between people in a relationship, may it be superficial or deep and long-lasting. In every relationship there are joys, sorrows, irritations and maybe some anger and disagreements. The disharmonious energies in a relationship create imbalances. In time the lack of harmony leads to even greater imbalances. An increasingly greater tension is built up between the individuals involved, and it becomes increasingly difficult to find the way back to harmony and love. With the help of Reiki it is possible to harmoniously and very effectively influence a relationship between two people who do not get along, or where one party is afraid of or angry with the other. This may concern the employer and the employee, the dentist or doctor and the patient, parents and children, friends, or a couple in an intimate relationship to mention a few. The effect of working with Reiki on relationships can be remarkable.

Additional techniques include subtle communication with others over a long distance. It is also possible to communicate with beings who are not able to understand the spoken word, for example people under anesthesia or in a coma, babies and small children, retarded people, and animals.

Reiki can be sent to any existing energy pattern, and since the entire universe is made of energies it is possible to transmit Reiki to absolutely everything. Sending harmonious Reiki to an important meeting, a test or exam, an operation or a doctor's visit, a delivery, a flight or a holiday, long before the event occurs are just a few examples of how and what Reiki can be used for.

Being able to selectively work on one's own inner blockages, fears, phobias, traumas, addictions etc. might still be the most useful technique taught in the Second Degree. Previous accidents, deaths, painful experiences, ones own limitations, belief systems, and anything else creating a hold up, physical pain or grief, may be worked on. The energy is sent to the actual event in order to balance the emotional charge around the problem that is still held today. It is not necessary to remember the cause of the problem for the sending to work. Obviously it is not possible to change what has already been done, but by dissolving the emotional charge still remaining, it is possible to let go and move on. Dissolving blockages created earlier in life, and which might have been carried internally for many years, offer an immense relief to the body and is the foundation for all personal unfoldment. This technique is one of the most powerful, simple and effective methods for personal growth and development.

The student learns many unique and exciting techniques that will help him lead a more harmonious and aware life. The Second Degree offers an exciting journey through time and space which, when used correctly, will lead to further growth and expansion.

However, it is important to know that the degree of information and teaching given in the Second Degree seminar varies widely from Reiki Master to Reiki Master. Many Masters choose to teach only the basic principles of the seminar, neglecting many of the more advanced techniques. The Reiki Network has a set minimum level of teaching for each Reiki degree. For the Second Degree this comprises at least ten hours, i.e. two full or three part time days, to allow appropriate duration for lectures and practical exercises. The Second Degree includes one more attunement in order for the body to adjust to the three energy formulas, and for the techniques to effectively work. The attunement allows an increased energy flow through the hands, an increase of the body's energy frequencies and thus a further expansion of the aura. The awareness expands when the body's subtle energies start to vibrate at a faster speed, and further personal development is thereby initiated.

An increased flow of Reiki provides a greater effect of the treatments, but there is a limit to the speed with which the body is able to heal itself. A practitioner who has taken both the Reiki Degrees will radiate more energy, which will speed up the healing of the body even more, but only to a certain level. There is a limit where the body cannot heal faster than it already does. The practitioners degree of Reiki will dramatically influence the end result mainly in cases of serious illnesses and problems.

Anyone who has graduated from Reiki First Degree may move on to the Second Degree. We recommend leaving at least a month in between the seminars to allow the student to experience maximum benefit from the subtle changes and new opportunities initiated by Reiki. Some students want to move on as fast as possible but many wait for a year or longer before continuing, while others remain content with their First Degree Reiki.

THIRD DEGREE—3A FOR PERSONAL GROWTH

The Third Degree—3A, spans over three days, totaling at least fifteen hours, but eighteen to twenty hours is preferable. This seminar has been developed as an intermediate level between the Second Degree and the Reiki Master training, but it is in fact a free-standing part of the Master training. Many people today have a need to explore themselves, increase their understanding, and to grow as individuals and spiritual beings. The 3A seminar offers an exceptionally effective opportunity to discover oneself.

The 3A seminar makes it possible to go further in Reiki and ones own development at a lower cost, both economically and personally, than what the Reiki Master training requires. Despite this, there are only a few people who are ready for the growth process initiated by the 3A seminar. Each person wanting to attend will first have to go through an interview to establish suitability. The Reiki Master Teacher will decide whether the time and occasion is right. In many instances it might be better for the person to wait with the 3A seminar and first establish the energy from the first two seminars before continuing. The Third Degree is not a short-cut to unfoldment and growth. The

First and Second Degrees must first be assimilated, the techniques used and results achieved before there can be any question of continuing to the next level. There should be at least six months and preferably up to a year or longer between the Second Degree and 3A.

In the 3A seminar the participants receive yet another attunement. The body's energy vibrations are further heightened, more Reiki radiates from the hands, the aura expands, and the opportunity for development increases dramatically. The attunement during the 3A seminar is very special. It affects the body and its subtle energies so powerfully that change and growth become inevitable. Old belief systems, prejudices, attitudes and lifestyles which are no longer relevant surface to make themselves remembered. This process makes it possible both to appropriately deal with and to finally release what is revealed. Human beings are often stuck in beliefs long since obsolete, founded as far back as early childhood. This rigid conditioning blocks and prevents us from living life fully, and to be present in the here and now. Instead we live at half speed while the rest of our energy is spent on following old belief systems and rigid opinions. Many of the challenges and joys of life are lost in the process. To be able to continue and allow ourselves to change we have to learn to release old habitual patterns that no longer serve a purpose. The 3A seminar is an effective step in accelerating the natural process of releasing.

The students learn another energy formula, a symbol with a very comprehensive ability to transform Reiki and expand its use in all areas. The students learn how to give the first Reiki attunement to others. By giving this attunement Reiki is *temporarily* activated in the hands of the recipient, remaining for a few weeks before disappearing. The client thereby receives the temporary ability to treat himself, and to experience Reiki first hand. The attunement is a very powerful treatment, which together with Reiki effectively supports the body's natural healing ability. Sick people benefit immensely from this combination. They can also treat themselves in between their appointments with the Third Degree practitioner. The energy emission from the hands ceases after a few weeks since all four attunements, each one different from the other, are required in order for Reiki to be permanently established in the body. Activating Reiki in others is a great responsibility, since the 3A practitioner is also lifting these people's awareness to a higher level.

Each time a 3A practitioner attunes another person to Reiki he too receives an attunement. The energy vibrations of both the recipient and the performer are strengthened and the awareness stimulated. This occurs each time an attunement is done. The opportunities for growth and expansion in somebody working with Reiki at this level are hereby endless. This is why the 3A is called the seminar for personal growth.

A 3A practitioner can also give booster attunements to people who already have Reiki. A process that by no means is necessary for the student to keep his Reiki, but which acts as an extra energy boost and as a potent treatment in conjunction with Reiki. The 3A practitioner often gives attunements at the group Reiki meetings. The attunement provides an extra energy supply, on top of the energy received in the group treatment.

The Reiki Alliance does not officially accept the 3A seminar as a degree. Its members will instead move their students straight from the Second Degree to the Master training which thereby becomes their Third Degree. The Reiki Master training is therefore called 3B to avoid misunderstandings and a mix up with students who have only gone as far as 3A.

T.R.T. has developed many more intermediate degrees including both 3A and 3B. They also separate some of their ensuing degrees in A and B.

The Reiki Network and many other associations and independent Reiki Masters adhere to the 3A Degree as an appropriate intermediate degree in between the Second Degree and Reiki Master training.

THE REIKI MASTER TRAINING

A Reiki Master is competent to teach First and Second Degree Reiki seminars. Though the duration and quality of the Master training varies immensely, from quick and superficial to thorough and lengthy. The price of the Master training varies in the same way. A higher price might suggest a more substantial education of a higher quality, and subsequently a greater end-result.

A few practitioners will move further, applying to be taken on for the Reiki Master training. Even fewer choose Reiki as a full-time occupation after graduation. Many Reiki Masters work with Reiki in their spare time giving only a few small seminars a year. This is one of the reasons why Reiki still is relatively unknown in our society. There are simply not enough well-educated Reiki Masters around having the confidence to promote themselves and Reiki. The more thorough the training the better equipped the Master will be after graduation when having to rely on himself and his knowledge.

A thorough Reiki Master training lasts a minimum of nine to twelve months in order to allow the student appropriate time to assimilate his own growth and to develop his work with the energies. Each part of the training requires new insights and changes in the student's energy vibrations and personality. The process forces the student to become aware of his own blockages and limitations, and to work through them. During the training period the student learns to perform a total of five different attunements. The student will learn each attunement by practical experience, i.e. he or she has to adopt and digest its deeper meaning, thereby achieving a higher degree of personal unfoldment. For this process to be successful it has to be allowed appropriate time.

Each initiation procedure involves an attunement of specific Chakras. While learning these attunements every one of them will initiate revolutionary processes within the student, which in turn will lead to deeper understanding and increased wisdom. The most important part of the training is the student's own growth, which must be allowed to take the time required. For most people this process takes approximately one year, though some students go through changes and development at a somewhat faster or slower pace. If this metamorphosis of the personality is not allowed to take place due to a too short period of training, the graduated Reiki Master will be unable to lift and expand other peoples awareness sufficiently. Instead he becomes an attunement technician while the deeper meaning of the initiation process will remain a mystery.

One first has to face and deal with ones own blockages, suppressed traumas, emotions and belief systems, before being able to awake another person's awareness to his problem areas, and the means to deal with what he encounters.

The Reiki Network's training of Reiki Masters is following a set manual, and runs over a minimum period of twelve months. The student has to take a number of oral assignments, which means intensive studies of different subjects. The assignments are presented to the Master Teacher either personally or by audio or video tapes. The tapes are corrected by the teacher who is also giving appropriate feed back. The student is expected to continue his endeavors until the teacher is completely satisfied that the student has reached at least the minimum standard set by the association. The training also includes a number of modules, evenly distributed over the year, where the teacher and students meet in person. These meetings include intensive training, practical exercises and group discussions. The students are also asked to sit in on First and Second Degree seminars given by the Master Teacher to learn in practice how the training is conducted. A large part of the training is done by correspondence.

Today many of the established Reiki associations require one year of training for new Reiki Masters, but the intensity, actual training, time schedule and content can still vary substantially. Unfortunately, there are certain individuals who choose to train others to the Reiki Master level during crash courses, sometimes as short as a weekend or a week. Both quality, seminars and confidence in Reiki will obviously suffer from this approach.

REIKI MASTER TEACHER—REIKI GRAND MASTER

A Reiki Master Teacher or Grand Master has furthered his education, and is qualified to give 3A seminars and train new Reiki Masters to the Master Teacher Degree. When a Reiki Master is regularly giving First and Second Degree seminars, and is actively working with Reiki, he or she is slowly growing into the energy of a Reiki Master. It is important that this process is not sped up or made too short. Once again it is a question of the Master's own development, and the releasing of old blockages, before it is appropriate to move on. The energy has to be established, and the Reiki Master needs time to assimilate the high vibrations he is working in. This development phase takes at least two years of dedicated work, and it often takes three years or longer before the Master qualifies for the Master Teacher Degree. The Master Teacher in charge of the training decides if and when the time to advance has arrived. A Reiki Master who is not actively giving seminars has no reason to move on to this next level of training. It is working with the Reiki energy that prepares the Master for the next degree. To a large extent the work conducted by the Master provides the further training.

A Master Teacher has reached as far as is possible within Reiki. Despite this, some Reiki associations and Masters have not let go of the idea that there has to be a particular successor and leading Grand Master in the world. Initially this might have been the tradition, but more than likely not. What ever the case, Hawayo Takata did never officially name any particular successor. The Reiki Alliance early on elected Phyllis Lei Furumoto, Hawayo Takata's Grand daughter, as the succeeding Grand Master. They are calling other Grand Masters for Master/Teachers in order to distinguish them from Phyllis. T.R.T. claims that their chairwoman, Barbara Webber Ray, is the world's leading Reiki Grand Master. The Reiki Network claims, among many independent Reiki Masters and other associations, that all Grand Masters are equal since they have reached the same level of degree and perform the same work. They are called either Reiki Master Teachers or Reiki Grand Masters according to their own choice.

PERSONAL REFLECTIONS

The length and thoroughness of the education of Reiki Masters is significant for it impacts the quality of the seminars the Master will conduct. Hence, a Master in training must understand the importance of his/her own unfoldment as an important part of the quality and content of the seminars to come. The Trainee must spend considerable time and effort on personal growth in order to attain the capability to initiate the same phase of growth in others. After all, being a Master means knowing how to master ones own life. If that is not achieved, at least to some degree, the Reiki Master will have little to offer others. A Reiki Master with only a short training is really nothing more than an attunement technician, in comparison with an established Reiki Master who has the ability to initiate people into new insights and heightened awareness.

There are crash courses in Reiki both for the First and Second Degrees, as well as for the 3A and Master training. There are Reiki Masters who do not seem to worry about giving both First and Second Degree seminars in consecutive order during the same weekend, allowing only one day for each seminar. The chance of successfully activating Reiki in an adult in one single day is slim. The time-span between the attunements is too short, and there is a great risk these people will not benefit from Reiki when the process is accelerated in this way. Worse even, some Masters state they have "modernized" Reiki, giving only one combined attunement during the seminar instead of the four traditional initiations. The participants on these courses might simply lose their Reiki after a while! The 3A seminar is also known to have some interesting variations, where the students might not receive neither their Master initiation nor learn how to perform the first attunement.

For those of you who want to have the Reiki energy activated in your hands it is worthwhile to check up on the Reiki Master and the contents of the seminar in advance. The length of the seminar also says something about the quality. A cheap one-day seminar may eventually become more expensive when it later turns out that the participants have not received the attunements correctly and thus has not had Reiki activated permanently. If this is the case further payment to attend a seminar by another Master will be necessary in order to permanently activate the energy.

Also the Reiki Master training may be carried out in the same irresponsible way, where a weekend or a few weeks are all that is given for the entire program. A person who believes he has struck a bargain by quickly going through the training at a lower cost and shorter time will soon realize the mistake. The standard of the seminars taught by such a quickie Master are of course inferior, the material insignificant and the attunements weak if at all correct. It will be difficult for this Master to attract participants to his seminars since his own energies are still in chaos. It is a simple fact that nobody who has not yet given himself time to develop will be able to expand other people's awareness. There is a big difference between an attunement technician, and a Master with experience and understanding of the inner esoteric depths of universal dynamics and psyche. A well-trained Reiki Master initiates a new beginning, a new future and new possibilities to his students. An attunement technician might (hopefully) activate Reiki in the hands of the participants. The difference is obviously significant.

My personal opinion is that it is worthwhile to attend seminars with a Reiki Master who has spent time and effort on his education. Not only because the contents of the seminar will be more comprehensive, but also because the process of the participants personal development and inner understanding is definitely initiated. For your own sake, I feel an absolute need to check on the Reiki Master's background and training as well as the length and contents of the seminar before you decide where and with whom you want to do your First Degree of Reiki. The general rule would apply here as well as anywhere else in society: you usually get what you pay for.

NINE

PEOPLE'S ENCOUNTERS WITH REIKI AND THEIR OWN STORIES

// *I want to share the following with you Lena because I can think of no one else I would wish to share these thoughts with more."*

This was the beginning of a letter to me from Maria, one of my Reiki students in New Zealand, and it continued like this:

"September 1992 you initiated me in Reiki and wonderful things began to happen. Actually it all began happening two weeks before being initiated. Course money and dates fell into the most perfect time frame. Having done another form of hands on healing Reiki felt equally good if not better. I am only sorry now that I did not keep some sort of a journal to record occurrences, for they were so many. My whole lifestyle changed dramatically because accepting the responsibility for my own health had a marvelous overspill into other areas of my life, for example, my creativity, connection and clairvoyance deepened. Previous to Reiki my life felt segregated, there were distinct areas and needless boundaries. Now I operate personally on an integrated level, things are clearer and easier. I do not compromise myself or feel the need to balance events. Reiki for me was and still is extremely personal and I did not give any treatments to others, apart from Reiki evenings, my partner and mother. This was not a deliberate rule but an instinctive act of attending to myself first before attempting to help heal others. I do not believe my work will be solely as a Reiki practitioner. Reiki is extremely important to me but it is not my life, it sheds light on my life."

"*Reiki, although completely separate from TM, seems to complement the meditation which I find terrific and learnt some years ago now. I do not need to consciously think positive, I am naturally more positive. I am out of so many personal traps that I still see others around me are in. Relationships have all moved on and as a result some of them have moved off completely. A wonderful purge occurred and freeing up of situations. Habitual cleanses and purges continue naturally when needed.*"

"*Art is another tool I have rediscovered. I paint, draw and sculpt whenever possible. I have put university on hold for another year or so because I have more perspective and respect in choosing what to learn. I have always been self-reliant, but now I am definitely more self responsible.*"

"*I am now a Freelancer putting all my skills from professional floristry to secretarial to use, managing to retain my independence and earn a decent living. For years I have fought with myself over what to do, my problem being not of "what" but "which" thing to do. I thought it was a curse to have such a variety of skills because it prevented me from being focused on a particular career. Now I laugh at this misguided belief caused by years of negative conditioning. Now I do everything I want, feeling very focused and happy.*"

"*I have nothing but respect for you Lena, and others like you, who devote their time and energy into bringing Reiki to others, it's wonderful.*"

I receive many letters similar to the one you have just read, and I have really understood the strength and depth of Reiki through my students' many experiences. It is with great respect and humility that I share my students' often very personal experiences, and the development and positive change the initiation of Reiki has brought to these people. Reiki is strongly affecting our personal development, but also other areas of our lives and health. I received this letter from Lena:

"The greatest thing Reiki and I have done together is absolutely my quitting smoking! I have now been smoke free for four months. I would never have made it without Reiki. I have previously made half-hearted attempts which have failed. Even this attempt was rather half-hearted to begin with, but I made it, thanks to Reiki."

"The strangest thing is that I don't have any problems with others who smoke. I don't get any mad cravings to smoke myself. Those feelings passed quite quickly. It was almost hardest when I was alone, but then I took help of my hands. More than a month has passed since I last craved a cigarette."

"This is how it happened: I have tried to give myself my Reiki hour every day. I later realized my hands rested on my solar plexus when I woke up in the morning. I therefore held my hands there when ever I had a chance during the day, for instance in the car, at work, in front of the TV, etc. I readily admit I didn't ponder upon why, I just felt that it was right. Later, when repeating your seminar, it clicked. Personal strength is located in the solar plexus. That's right! That's how it is. That is exactly what I need not to have a cigarette when the craving is so bad."

"In addition to Reiki I have also worked with a home-made mixture of meditation, relaxation and affirmations. I have done this during my Reiki hour. I have gone to my inner place as you taught us in the seminar, and I have told myself that I don't smoke. I believe the need to smoke depends to a degree on the image one has of oneself as a smoker, and if one manages to change that picture it is easier to quit."

"Reiki has done a lot for me, and sometimes I wonder how much Reiki is a way of life, and how much it is an aid to experience more? It really doesn't matter, but sometimes I wonder.... Reiki has definitely helped me see life in a brighter light. For many years I have worked on trying to see the positive things in life, and it has been substantially easier since I have started to use Reiki. I don't take things as seriously any longer."

"I have also started to see auras around some people's heads. That is pretty cool. I start with looking around wondering whether the sun is shining through a window and thus creating the light effect. Then I wonder if it is the reflection from something else before I finally realize that it is actually a shining light around the person's head that I am seeing."

Reiki has no limitations, and it provides us with exactly what we need for the moment. The awareness expansion allows a better perception of subtle energies, for instance the ability to see the auric fields radiating from all living beings. Reiki also moves us deeper in contact with our own psyche and physical environment. One of my female students wrote the following in her letter:

"I got a better marriage when my spiritual strength grew with Reiki. Just daring to move on to the outer limb and see what has gone wrong over the years, then using the soothing effects of Reiki to mend the errors in us both. This has been very educating, and we now pass this knowledge on to others."

The positive psychological effect of Reiki can be remarkable. Katharina tells the story of how she helped a woman out of her severe depression by applying repeated Reiki treatments. This is her story:

"Mia came to me in September after recommendations from her partner. She was very depressed, and had been unable to work for the past six months because of her depression. She had no strength, was lethargic, and didn't really believe in life getting any better. Reiki was just another attempt to break out of the depression. She was also seeing a psychologist regularly."

"During the first week Mia came for three treatments, and thereafter twice a week. After the fourth treatment Mia had an appointment with her psychologist. The first words the psychologist said when seeing Mia was how wonderful it was to see she had once more started to live, how vital she looked, and that there now was a light in her eyes. The psychologist prescribed continued Reiki treatments. Mia started to

activate herself. She began exercising her body, enjoying her child, and she felt less reluctance in taking care of her home. She also began to look for a new education that would lead to a job she could enjoy."

"The last time I treated Mia was in the middle of March. By then she was full of inspiration and in anticipation of the new education she was to start a month later. She had had a hair-cut, and she had begun to wear clothes in different colors instead of, as previously, only black. She was also keeping herself busy with several projects at home."

Ingela from the south of Sweden wrote the following:

"I feel much better, and I have a totally different view on life and myself since learning Reiki. I feel joy and harmony within myself. I no longer become angry over little things, and those around me are also behaving differently towards me. I have become more open towards everybody, and many more people are coming to me with their small or big problems. They say they feel a certain strength in me. Reiki has made it much more easy to understand why we sometimes feel as we do. I feel like I am a new person."

"I was the one who had chocolate cysts, or endometriosis. I was on medication for over five years for this, but after the Reiki seminar and a sacri-cranial treatment I haven't taken any medication at all. I have done one hour of Reiki every day since the seminar, and at the gynecological examination a month and a half later the doctor could not find one single cyst! Everything feels wonderful now!"

Physical healing of the body is one of the great benefits of Reiki. The following story was given to me by a woman who had worked with Reiki First Degree for a few months when the event occurred:

"Calle was close to ninety years old, but lived at home and took care of himself until one day when he was admitted to hospital due to stomach pains. He had a high temperature and it was established that Calle had an abscess at the pancreas. He was treated with antibiotics but was still in pain."

"The weeks passed. Calle's fever fits came and went despite different cures of antibiotics, and he started to grow weaker. From initially being able to walk about, he was now bed-ridden. When I visited Calle he was virtually convulsing from fever shivers—as usual. I suddenly became so upset, wishing for him to be free of these taxing fever tops. I screened off the bed, sat down and put my hands over his pancreas. Calle was hardly aware of my presence, but he could feel my "warm nice hands". I sat with my hands on Calle's abdomen for approximately twenty minutes, and then I went home. Imagine my surprise when I, a couple of days later, found out that Calle was on his way home. The X-rays showed that the abscess was gone—finally, after several weeks of struggling with different cures of antibiotics. Consequently Calle was also free of fever. I was not the only one who stood gaping at this turn of events!"

Through Reiki we may experience many almost miraculous healings both of body and mind, but Reiki only heals if we are ready to let go of our dis-ease. To start with, we may have to remember, or realize from where, and why the problem arose.

Pelle, who is approximately thirty-five years old, had suffered serious back-problems all of his adult life. The back-pains forced Pelle to go on sick-leave for longer and longer periods. During the first four to five years his sick-leaves lasted for days and weeks up to a month at a time, but soon the convalescence lasted for a month or more. Various specialists stood powerless, and he was not admitted to the special back-clinic since his problems were considered too severe. After ten years of chronic and very severe pains, and long periods of sick-leave, Pelle could no longer continue his physically demanding job. The doctors recommended Pelle to re-train for a new career.

Pelle came into contact with Reiki almost fifteen years after his severe back-pains begun. He immediately went through an intense phase of ten to fifteen long and frequent treatments. He slept through the first few treatments, and was totally shaken by the energy he experienced. Later, when awake and more aware, he experienced the treatments even more powerfully. In the beginning of the treatment period he felt a dreadful jerking and pulling in the chest area over the heart, but after a number of treatments he just felt nice and relaxed.

Occasionally Pelle had to have emergency treatments for his severe pains. Initially the pains increased as a result of the treatment, and then subsided after approximately twelve hours. After a couple of months of regular Reiki treatments, Pelle re-lived a very difficult personal experience which had taken place in his teens, and had been suppressed since then. This time he was able to allow himself to release all the pain and grief that he had previously buried, and which had been stored in the body ever since then. He now understood how this event, which had not been sufficiently dealt with as a teenager, was the root cause of all his back-pains. After this episode Pelle experienced an enormous joy and relief. He had finally managed to let go of his difficult experience, and was able to get on with life. Pelle's back-pains have almost vanished since then. If he happens to feel a twitch from his back he uses Reiki and meditation to heal. Of course it goes without saying that Pelle learned Reiki for himself as soon as he had the opportunity.

Pelle was unable to heal until he became aware of the strong hold the suppressed teenage trauma had over his life today. He had to release all the grief and pain which had been pushed into his body so many years ago when he was unable to deal with the event. It was not possible to let go of the pain in the back until he had re-lived and worked through this experience. In other cases it might not be necessary for old memories to surface, and consciously be worked through. It happens just as often that suppressed experiences are dealt with on a deeper level beyond words and conscious thoughts. Then the body takes care of the difficult past experience without revealing any particular images or memories. This was the case for Yvonne.

Yvonne had had problems with her back and neck for almost fifteen years when she attended one of my First Degree seminars. She had previously tried both acupuncture and physiotherapy but achieved no results. Her entire right side was in pain and she was unable to stand on one leg without losing her balance. One month after the seminar Yvonne phoned to tell me about her improvements. She was astonished that the only remnants of her back and neck problems were a light pain between her shoulder blades! Apart from this her mind was clearer, both mentally and spiritually. Her bad stomach was better and the constipation gone, she suffered less from PMS and was in a better mood during her period. Yvonne exclaimed delightedly that all this had happened in a month. She could hardly wait to see what would happen in a year.

Children too are experiencing Reiki very positively, especially when hurting themselves. Christina's seven year old son Patrick happened to put his arm over the toaster. He immediately received a third degree burn and developed an open wound. Around the wound the arm was red and burnt on an area larger than the palm of Christina's hand. Christina immediately put his arm in cold water and then gave several Reiki applications, approximately twenty to thirty minutes in total. In less than two hours the red area around the burn was completely gone. The burn itself developed a crust and healed extremely fast without complications. Patrick was never in pain despite the fact that the clothes often grated the wound. When the burn had healed it did not even leave a scar! Today it is impossible to see that his arm was once badly burnt.

I would like to add that it is possible to treat burns with Reiki at the same time as the injured area is cooled under running water or dipped in a bucket of ice-water.

By accident John's fifteen year old nephew Michael was hit in the eye by a fire-cracker. Michael was urgently taken to the hospital where the pressure in the eye was measured in connection with the diagnosis. Normal eye pressure would be around 15 kgp, but the pressure in Michael's eye measured 55 kgp. The doctor feared Michael would lose his sight but could do nothing more than dress the eye and send him home. When Michael came home from the hospital tears were pouring from the injured eye, the pupil was very small and he could not open his eye. John was urgently sent for, and he gave Michael plenty of Reiki. The next day Michael could open the eye, the pupil was of normal size and his perfect sight was intact.

Patrice wrote a letter to me where she tells of how she experienced her first contact with Reiki and what happened later:

"My first introduction to Reiki was through my parents who had done Reiki I (First Degree) in their home country. They were extremely enthusiastic about it, even my very skeptical father."

"Several months later I saw an advertisement in our local news paper for a free public Reiki lecture. Being a scientist with what I call "an open mind", I went along to satisfy my curiosity. I thoroughly enjoyed your lecture Lena. Your "down to earth" approach focusing on practical matters, and your science degree in agriculture gave a lot of credibility in my eyes."

"Coming home from this lecture I told my (extremely skeptical) husband that I didn't know whether to believe in it or not but that I would love to try First Degree Reiki. The whole thing seemed too good to be true, but I said that I still wanted to try it. The only problem was: money. That same evening my mother rang from Holland, completely out of the blue. I told her about my brush with Reiki. She was very enthusiastic and offered to pay for my seminar."

"The very next Reiki First Degree seminar saw me participate eagerly. It was the most amazing experience, I would never be the same again. My hands were burning, I saw bolts of light shafting through my body during the attunements. I found it hard to accept all these things in contrast to some of the other participants who took to it like a fish to water."

"Life was different after Reiki I. I was full of energy and felt almost constantly "on a high". The most noticeable thing was that I (an absolute coffee addict) couldn't stand the taste of coffee."

"There was no doubt in my mind that I wanted to do Reiki II (Second Degree Reiki) This seminar was totally different from the first. I spent most of my time writing furiously. So much fantastic information, I couldn't bare to miss any of it. Some of the stuff went way over my head, some of the stuff I couldn't cope with (I am not at all a spiritual person). However, that didn't matter as there was no great emphasis on spiritual things."

"The weeks after this seminar I felt extremely tired. I slept far more than usual. And I couldn't help feeling a bit disappointed that I didn't feel the same exhilaration as after Reiki I. I joined the group Reiki sessions and that was a good move. To be able to talk to like minded people is very important if you go through a period of change."

"I had set out to "heal the world". There were many people in my environment that "needed some help". At least that was what I decided. In no time at all I had completely exhausted myself. Of course the Reiki group had been kept up to date with my experiences and they had been warning me for this "burnout", but you have to experience these things for yourself. I understood now that my tiredness was caused by me sacrificing my own Reiki treatments in order to have time to help everybody else. I spent the next couple of weeks sending only to myself. And since then I have mainly treated only my family and myself."

"I then "sat in" on another Reiki II seminar which I found very helpful. Many things made more sense to me now that I had had a bit of practice. Especially the bit of looking after yourself!"

"My husband didn't know what to think of it all. He was very skeptical, but also very pleased that Reiki did so much good for me. He noticed that I could handle far more stress than usual. Falling asleep had been a problem for me for many years, now I just "send" myself to sleep."

"Having a full time teaching job, two kids and a husband overseas for a few weeks, as well as trying to sell your house is an incredible load for any one. I would not have been able to do it without all the Reiki I have sent and given to myself every day. Headaches, tummy aches, tiredness, cuts, bruises and blisters, all disappear or become bearable with Reiki. Even my skeptical husband has had his back fixed by Reiki recently. Although he still maintains it might have been just a nice "coincidence". It is amazing how many "nice coincidences" we have had in this household in the last year!"

Patrice has treated many people and she continues like this:

"The fastest result I have obtained was with Rita (the sister of a friend of mine). I knew that she suffered from ME (chronic fatigue-syndrome) for the last two years. She was very weak and felt very depressed. One evening my friend (whom I had told all about my Reiki experiences) rang me and asked me to come over and see her sister, who was staying with her at that time. Rita was going through a very bad patch. So I eagerly set out on my mission."

"I had a chat with Rita and explained all about Reiki. Then I gave her a one hour hands-on treatment. The area around the neck was very sensitive and Rita couldn't stand my hands there at all (too hot). At the end of the treatment, she had developed a heat rash on her throat and upper chest. And I hadn't even touched her there!"

"Rita felt very relaxed and sleepy and went to bed, and I went home. The next day my friend rang me to say that Rita had felt a lot better and had gone back home. I sent Reiki to Rita three times that week and once a week the following couple of weeks. The results were amazing. Rita rang me a couple of times to report on her progress. Within a month she was painting her room, had taken on a part-time job, and was planning a holiday to Australia. She hadn't felt this good for a long, long time!"

Reiki can be just as effective when sent over a distance, as when the energy is transferred through a physical hands on treatment. Helena told me about Margareta, a woman who unsuccessfully had tried to become pregnant for several years. Since the two women lived far apart, Helena offered to send Reiki to Margareta. Helena sent the first Reiki treatment on the fourth of November, and continued to send Reiki once a week thereafter. Margareta called around Christmas to say that she suspected she was pregnant. The first weekend after Christmas her suspicions were confirmed. Margareta happily told Helena that she was really pregnant. Little Elin was born in late summer, and Helena says it feels like she is part of the joyful event.

Absentee Reiki can be used for so much more than healing of the physical body. It is as easy to heal emotional traumas as balancing future events. Anna tells me she uses the First Degree technique on her body every morning when giving herself one hour of Reiki. She also sends Reiki regularly to the past in order to heal and create harmony. Anna says she sends Reiki to future events too, and this has given her a sense of doing something useful without getting tangled in all sorts of unnecessary activity and repeating yet some more Karma. She seems to have dropped a lot of excess baggage this way, and she has also physically lost about seven kilos in weight. Anna says that she feels wonderful after all this Reiki.

Nellie, an elderly lady who has attended both the First and Second Degree seminars, sends Reiki every day to her family and friends, but also to many future events, such as exams, journeys, job applications, and meetings to improve communication. She also sends Reiki to all the wonderful new things she is learning and wishes to retain and use thoroughly, like her recent reading course and Reiki seminars. Nellie says that nowadays it is automatic to think: "I'll send Reiki to that!"

Animals and plants also benefit from Reiki. Sick animals often respond very quickly to treatments since they do not have as many blockages and hang ups as people. Monica sent me this story:

"I went to my riding lesson as usual on Friday. I was then told the horse of one of the employees at the stable was very sick, and I asked if I could try giving it Reiki. Titti, the owner of the horse, immediately agreed. That morning the horse's temperature had been 39,7o C. When

I started the treatment the temperature was 38,7o C. The legs of the horse were very swollen. The horse, who suffered from an infection of the lymph, loitered, nice as a lamb. I crawled around its legs holding them, as well as its shoulder. Finally I held my hands behind its "chin". The horse was thoroughly enjoying the treatment. After approximately twenty minutes, its belly rumbled so loudly it startled Titti. She had never heard anything like it. The horse passed wind every now and then during the treatment. Titti held the horse's head and after approximately forty minutes it tried to bite her arm. The horse started to grow restless and was sort of telling us that it didn't want to be part of this anymore. I quickly ran out of the box, and Titti exclaimed happily that the horse was as mean as usual again! The horse was given its evening hay, ate contentedly, and was cheeky. Titti called the next morning to tell me the horse had no temperature, and that the swelling of the legs was completely gone. You can imagine how happy I was!"

I get to hear many wonderful stories about animals, and it is a joy to see how much we seem to care about our animals and how much they benefit from Reiki. I was told about a cat that had been run over so badly it couldn't move its hind quarters at all. It was able to move slightly only by dragging itself forward with the help of its front legs. The cat loved its Reiki sessions, and its injuries healed very quickly. It still returns frequently for more Reiki despite its complete recovery.

Maria writes: *"A cat ill with cancer, complete with weeping welts, transformed into a happy cat with shining ginger fur and no sign of sickness. Successful cures and easier passing for animals with terminal illnesses have occurred. My three cats, two of which were adopted from an animal shelter having survived serious neglect and cruelty, are a picture of good health and joy."*

Also trees, bushes, flowers, and all other living things grow and flourish when receiving an extra supplement of Reiki. Maria also writes about a dying tree destined for the ax that, one week later and after only two sessions of Reiki, was a total mass of flowers and bright green foliage.

Gerd gave Reiki to the bag of seeds before planting the seeds in her vegetable garden. When autumn arrived she was able to harvest beet-roots of 1.5 kilos.

Reiki balances the energies of all living beings and increases the inherent healing power within, but the wonders of Reiki extends far beyond biological matter. It has been shown that even so-called inanimate objects may benefit from Reiki and repair themselves. Sylvia sent this story to me:

"One day in June I visited a seventy-six year old lady at her house deep in the forest. The woman lives alone far from any other people or services, and she is only able to move with difficulty. Her brother passed away the previous spring, and nobody had been cutting the grass around her cottage this summer. To my astonishment I was told the grass had always been cut with a scythe, and that modern inventions weren't all that welcome. Since using a scythe is an art that I have never learned to master, I suggested that I would go and get my own lawn-mover to help her make it look nice around her cottage. The lady then told me there was in fact an old lawn-mover which had been standing in the barn for the last eight years. It had been inherited from an older brother who had passed away many years ago. I got the old, rusty lawn-mover out and to my surprise I found there was petrol in the tank. However the spark plugs were placed in a very awkward position and hard to get to. I wasn't able to take them out for cleaning. After laboriously pulling the starting strap over and over I was ready to throw the rickety old thing back into the dust in the barn. That's when I got the idea. Give Reiki! I squatted down and with sweaty hands I gave the rusty old motor Reiki. In the meantime I told the old lady about Reiki's incredible effect on all living things. Since she had received Reiki from me several times she thought it would be exciting to see whether the lawn-mover was susceptible as well. After a few minutes of Reiki I once again pulled the strap, and the motor started! We cried with astonishment and couldn't believe our eyes. The lawn-mower worked as well as anything, and I mowed the lawn around her little cottage while feeling a humble respect for the wonderful power of Reiki."

Bo was riding a snow scooter when he experienced the following:

"It was a wonderful moonlit evening with calm weather. We turned off our snow scooters for a while to enjoy the quiet night. When about to continue our journey the starting strap didn't catch in the cogs, it rather behaved like a rubber-band. My friend claimed it would be necessary to repair the scooter, and began preparing to tow it home. I said I wanted to try some Reiki on the starter. I gave Reiki for a few minutes and then tried again. Nothing happened. I sat for a few more minutes. At the next try all of a sudden the cogs caught and the snow scooter started. We have no technical explanation for this."

Birgitta had the opportunity to show what Reiki is capable of when about to do some photo-copying. She relates the following:

"When I came into the copy room a young man was already there, angrily cursing the photocopier which wasn't working. I told him I would give the machine some Reiki. The boy looked indulgently at me, almost thinking aloud that I must be absolutely out of my mind. I carefully placed my hands on the machine and stood like that for a few minutes. To the boy's great astonishment the machine started, and he left without saying word."

Reiki is a wonderful method of making life easier for everyone choosing to work with the technique. All that is needed is four attunements for the Reiki energy to be activated in the body systems. This is done during a two-day First Degree Reiki seminar. Reiki is not only bringing about optimal health, but also personal development and growth, inner understanding, and a deeper connection with life. Humans, animals, plants and objects are all positively affected by Reiki and its ability to create harmony, balance and health in everything touched by its wonder.

I wish you much luck in making your own choice. If choosing Reiki, you will be sure to have a gift for life. A gift that will help you through many difficult times, problems and dis-eases.

I want to conclude this book with a few lines from one of my Reiki students. She writes:

"Reiki to me is much more than treating myself and others for preventive or physical healing purposes. Reiki means the possibility to understand, and also to cope, with life itself."

SEMINAR INFORMATION

For seminar information in different countries see:
www.reikinetwork.com

ORDERS

Following items may be ordered:

SADHANA—FOR REIKI AND RELAXATION
CD or tape

Sadhana—the path to love, is deeply relaxing music in twelve parts, each five minutes long, that gently guides you through a Reiki session. Acoustic guitar, keyboards, and various wind instruments, interwoven with the healing sounds of nature, invite you on a relaxing inner journey. Each track ending with soft wind chimes. A popular best seller.

HOMECOMING—MEDITATIVE MUSIC FOR REIKI, RELAXATION AND HEALING
CD only

Homecoming, twelve five minute pieces of beautiful music ideal for a Reiki treatment. The haunting sound of the loon, rainforest birds of Australia, sounds from the depth of the earth, all combined with spellbinding music that creates the perfect environment for deep relaxation and stress release. Each track ending with the light bell sound of Tibetan Ting Sha's.

DEEP WATERS
Tape only

Soothing ocean sounds recorded in different locations around New Zealand's beautiful coastline. This tape contains twelve tracks of five minute duration, with a gentle bell between each to lead you through a Reiki treatment. Let yourself relax to the different moods of the Pacific Ocean and the unique coastal environment.

ORDER FROM:

Energy for Life AB
Att: Peter Forster
c/o Blabärsvägen 2
S-774 62 Avesta
Sweden
E-mail: pforster@swipnet.se

Another excellent source of Reiki and Therapeutic Music is:
Inner Worlds Music
P.O. Box 325
Twin Lakes, WI 53181
USA.
They may be contacted at:
Toll Free: 800 444 9678
Website: www.innerworldsmusic.com
E-mail: innerworlds@lotuspress.com

INDEX

Abrasions 90

Absentee Reiki 125, 148

Addiction 125, 127

Affirmation 18, 49, 126, 139

AIDS (Acquired Immune Deficiency
  Syndrome) 13, 24

A.I.R.A. (American International Reiki
  Association) 121

Anger 17, 23, 33-34, 41, 53, 64, 67, 80,
  116, 126

Animals 42, 43, 113-114, 126, 148, 149,
  151

A.R.A. (American Reiki Association) 121

Armor 56-58, 104

Astral body 17

Attunement 10-13, 15, 16, 28, 52, 79, 96,
  100, 103, 105, 114, 119, 120, 121,
  124, 127, 129, 130, 131, 132, 134,
  135, 145, 151
    booster 130

Aura 8, 9, 15-16, 19, 20, 21, 25, 29, 42,
  114, 127, 129, 140

Back pain 97
  problems 142, 143

Belief systems 13, 19, 29, 30, 49, 52, 53,
  54, 58, 64, 125, 127, 129, 132

Bioplasm 8, 15

Blockages 16, 20, 22, 23, 24, 25, 30, 32,
  38, 59, 67, 87, 104, 127, 131, 132, 133,
  148

Blue light 92

Burns 90, 104, 144

Causal body 17, 19

Cells 8, 9, 29, 78, 111

Chakra major 17, 21-28, 85, 131
  first (root) 22, 25

second (sacral) 22-23, 25
  third (solar plexus) 23, 25
  fourth (heart) 23-24, 26, 28
  fifth (throat) 24, 26
  sixth (third eye) 25, 26
  seventh (crown) 25, 26

Chakra minor 28

Chakra system 27, 28, 31

Chakra treatment 126

Chi (Qi/Ki) 12,

Childhood 53, 55, 56, 58, 125, 129

Children 11, 34, 41, 46, 49, 50, 53, 55,
  91, 104-105, 126, 141, 144
    hyperactive 105

Chinese medicine 31-33

Chronic fatigue syndrome 147

Consciousness 4, 21, 27, 87, 125
  victim 63

Contra-indications 47, 48

Cuts 90, 104, 147

Depression 39-41, 51, 140

Destiny 17

Detachment 65-67, 72, 92-93

Detoxification 80

Diagnosis 43, 44, 47, 144

Diarrhea 80, 100

Disease 12, 16, 24, 29, 31, 32, 33, 38, 39,
  41, 42, 43, 45, 46, 48, 77, 87, 102,
  109, 110, 111, 152

Disturbance 9, 13, 16, 17, 27, 30, 44, 79,
  87

Education 6, 14, 44, 53, 60, 88, 99, 102,
  121, 122, 123, 131, 132, 133, 135, 141

Ego 20, 24, 25, 44, 49-52, 64, 74, 92, 93,
  102, 109
    centered 40

Endocrine glands 21, 22, 23, 24, 25, 27
Endocrine system 24, 31, 34
Ether body 19
Etheric body 8, 19-20
Fear 22, 24, 34-37, 41, 46, 53, 56, 61, 66, 69, 109, 125, 127
Fever 142
First-aid 48
First Degree 5, 11, 84, 96, 103, 122, 124, 128, 132, 133, 134, 135, 141, 143, 145, 148, 151
Freedom of choice 60
Frequencies 8, 9-10, 15, 20, 29, 44, 87, 103, 106, 125, 127
Furumoto, Phyllis Lei 120-121, 133
Gamma rays 9
GMO (gene modified organisms) 43
Grand Master 5, 120, 123, 132, 133
Gratitude 72, 73
Grief 38-39, 40, 41, 63, 64, 127, 143
Group Reiki 106-107, 130, 146
   treatment 106, 130
Hawaii 4, 5, 119
Hawkin, Stephen 10
Hayashi, Chujiro 4, 5
Headache 34, 71, 80, 93, 100, 146
Healing crisis 79, 100-101
   process 2, 7, 11, 13, 44, 45, 47, 79, 87, 89, 90, 94, 111, 124
Heller work 31
Higher self 50-52, 64, 74
HIV (Human Immunodeficiency Virus) 13, 24
Inanimate objects 118, 150
Initiation 10, 73, 131, 134, 138
   process 73, 132
Intuition 14, 20, 25, 26, 49, 74, 85, 93, 98, 102, 103
Joy 17, 19, 20, 33, 39-41, 51, 61, 63, 64, 66, 67, 76, 83, 124, 126, 129, 141,143, 149

Karma 109-110, 148
   debt 110
Life force 10-12, 37, 42, 115
Living spiritually 72
Lower self 49-51, 65, 78
Magnetic healing 98
Manipulate 58, 75
Manipulation 58, 76
Marathon Reiki 108
Masks 56-57
Meditation 3, 47, 87, 138, 139, 143
Mental body 19
Microwaves 9
Money 40, 83, 101, 118, 121, 137, 145
Monitor 122
Music 85, 98, 153
Nausea 34, 80, 100
Neck problem 143-144
Nerve 44
   complex 21, 22
   synapse 55
Observer the 65, 72
Organism 7, 9, 43
Pain 30-31, 34, 42, 46, 57, 63, 64, 66, 79-80, 82, 84, 89, 90, 93, 97, 100, 101, 102, 106, 110, 127, 141, 142-143, 144
   relief 46, 91, 104, 108, 109
Painful 30, 34, 57, 88, 100, 127
Particles 8, 9, 10, 13, 29
Personal growth 123, 127, 128, 130, 134
Phobia 125, 127
Plants 113, 114-115, 116, 148, 151
Polarity healing 98
Preventive 6, 14, 48, 77, 96, 124, 152
Quantum physics 8, 125
   physicists 9, 10
Radiance Technique the (T.R.T.) 121, 123, 130, 133
Rebirthing 31
Reiki Alliance the 120-121, 123, 130, 133

Reiki Grand Master 5, 120, 123, 132-133
Reiki Master 1, 6, 11, 52, 59, 96, 105, 119-123, 127, 128, 130-132, 133, 134, 135
    independent 121, 123, 130, 133
Reiki Master Teacher 121, 123, 128, 132-133
Reiki Network the 121-123, 127, 130, 132, 133
Relationships 23, 26-27, 51, 55, 57, 58, 64, 67-69, 78, 125, 126, 138
Relaxation 48, 85, 87-88, 90, 97, 98, 99, 139, 153
Responsibility 6, 16, 18, 20, 22, 53-54, 60, 65, 68, 72, 73, 88, 91, 92, 94, 96, 119, 130, 137
Roles 51, 56-58, 67
Rolfing 31
Rosen therapy 31
Sanskrit 3, 21
Second Degree 122, 123, 124-128, 129, 130, 132, 133, 134, 146, 148
Self esteem 18, 24, 55, 69
Self worth 45, 56, 64, 72, 76, 77, 102
Seminars information 158
Smoking 51, 91, 117, 139
Soul 19, 20, 23, 25, 41, 50-52, 64, 72, 110
    bodies 20
    searching 32
Speed of light 11, 125
Standard 45, 119, 120, 121, 122, 132, 135
Stress release 48, 88, 96, 153
Subconscious 18, 19, 20, 32, 49, 51, 54, 59, 78, 82, 101
Subtle anatomy 8, 9, 15-16, 28
Successor 4, 5, 6, 120, 133
Sumerians 1
Super-conscious 19, 20, 49, 50, 82
Supra luminal speed 9
Surrender 70-72, 73, 84, 92

Sutras 3
Symbols 3, 124
Symptoms 16, 29, 30, 32, 36, 38, 39, 41, 43, 48, 61, 77, 94, 101, 110
Tai Chi 47
Takata, Hawayo 4-5, 133
Theory of the five elements the 33
Third Degree—3A 123, 128, 129, 130, 132, 134
Training 5, 6, 14, 91, 119-123, 131, 132, 133, 134, 135
    manual 122, 132
    Master 121, 123, 128, 130-132, 133, 134, 135
    Master Teacher 132-133
Trauma 30, 42, 54, 98, 127, 132, 143, 148
Ulcer 37, 43-44
Unconscious 19, 30, 38, 51, 55, 88
Unfoldment 37, 47, 51, 73, 76, 127, 128, 131, 134
Unified Field Theory the 10
Universal life energy 1, 3, 10
Unpolarized energy 9, 11, 125
Usui, Mikao 2-4, 120
Veltheim, John & Esther 122
Visualize 93, 102
Worry 3, 37-38, 44, 66, 100, 101, 134
X-rays 9, 142
Yin and Yang 25-27, 67
Yoga 47

Herbs and other natural health products and information are often available at natural food stores or metaphysical bookstores. If you cannot find what you need locally, you can contact one of the following sources of supply.

Sources of Supply:

The following companies have an extensive selection of useful products and a long track-record of fulfillment. They have natural body care, aromatherapy, flower essences, crystals and tumbled stones, homeopathy, herbal products, vitamins and supplements, videos, books, audio tapes, candles, incense and bulk herbs, teas, massage tools and products and numerous alternative health items across a wide range of categories.

WHOLESALE:

Wholesale suppliers sell to stores and practitioners, not to individual consumers buying for their own personal use. Individual consumers should contact the RETAIL supplier listed below. Wholesale accounts should contact with business name, resale number or practitioner license in order to obtain a wholesale catalog and set up an account.

Lotus Light Enterprises, Inc.
P O Box 1008 RHP
Silver Lake, WI 53170 USA
262 889 8501 (phone)
262 889 8591 (fax)
800 548 3824 (toll free order line)

RETAIL:

Retail suppliers provide products by mail order direct to consumers for their personal use. Stores or practitioners should contact the wholesale supplier listed above.

Internatural
33719 116th Street RHP
Twin Lakes, WI 53181 USA
800 643 4221 (toll free order line)
262 889 8581 office phone
EMAIL: internatural@lotuspress.com
WEB SITE: www.internatural.com

Web site includes an extensive annotated catalog of more than 10,000 items that can be ordered "on line" for your convenience 24 hours a day, 7 days a week.

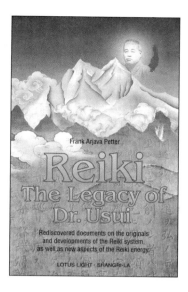

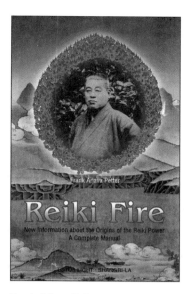

Frank Arjava Petter

Reiki – The Legacy of Dr. Usui

Rediscovered documents on the origins and developments of the Reiki system, as well as new aspects of the Reiki energy

A great deal has been written and said to date about the history of Reiki and his founder. Now Frank Ajarva Petter a Reiki Master who lives in Japan, has come across documents that quote Mikao Usui's original words. Questions that his students asked and he answered throw light upon Usui's very personal view of the teachings. Materials meant as the basis for his student's studies round off the entire work. A family tree of the Reiki successors is also included here. In a number of essays, Frank Ajarva Petter also discusses topics related to Reiki and the viewpoints of an independent Reiki teacher.

128 pages · $12.95
ISBN 0-914955-56-X

Frank Arjava Petter

Reiki Fire

New Information about the Origins of the Reiki Power A Complete Manual

The origin of Reiki has come to be surrounded by many stories and myths. The author, an independent Reiki Master practicing in Japan, immerses it in a new light as he traces Usui-san's path back through time with openness and devotion. He meets Usui's descendants and climbs the holy mountain of his enlightenment. Reiki, shaped by Shintoism, is a Buddhist expression of Qigong, whereby Qigong depicts the teaching of life energy in its original sense. An excellent textbook, fresh and rousing in its spiritual perspective, this is an absolutely practical Reiki guide. The heart, the body, the mind, and the esoteric background, are all covered here.

144 pages, $12.95
ISBN 0-914955-50-0

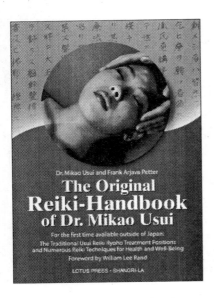

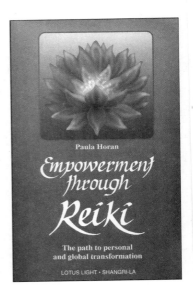

Dr. Mikao Usui and Frank A. Petter

The Original Reiki Handbook

The Traditional Usui Reiki Ryoho Treatment Positions and Numerous Reiki Techniques for Health and Well-Being

For the first time available outside of Japan: This book will show you the original hand positions from Dr. Usui's handbook. It has been illustrated with 100 colored photos to make it easier to understand. The hand positions for a great variety of health complaints have been listed in detail, making it a valuable reference work for anyone who practices Reiki. Now that the original handbook has been translated into English, Dr. Usui's hand positions and healing techniques can be studied directly for the first time. Whether you are an initiate or a master, if you practice Reiki you can expand your knowledge dramatically as you follow in the footsteps of a great healer.

80 pages, 100 photos, $ 14.95
ISBN 0-914955-57-8

Dr. Paula Horan

Empowerment Through Reiki

The Path to Personal and Global Transformation

In a gentle and loving manner, Dr. Paula Horan, world-renowned Reiki Master and bestselling author, offers a clear explanation of Reiki energy and its healing effects. This text is a must for the experienced practitioner. The reader is leaded through the history of this remarkable healing work to the practical application of it using simple exercises. We are not only given a deep understanding of the Reiki principles, but also an approach to this energy in combination with other basic healing like chakra balancing, massage, and work with tones, colors, and crystals. This handbook truly offers us personal transformation, so necessary for the global transformation at the turn of the millennium.

160 pages, $ 14.95
ISBN 0-941524-84-1